THE STATUS OF THE HUMAN EMBRYO

THE STATUS OF
THE HUMAN EMBRYO

Perspectives from moral tradition

Edited by
G R Dunstan and Mary J Seller

King Edward's Hospital Fund for London

© King Edward's Hospital Fund for London 1988
Printed and bound in England by Oxford University Press

Distributed for the King's Fund by Oxford University Press

ISBN 0 19 724644 3

King's Fund Publishing Office
14 Palace Court
London W2 4HT

CONTENTS

ACKNOWLEDGMENTS

Chapter 5 in this book is an expanded version of a submission in evidence to the Warnock committee, published in the *Journal of Medical Ethics*, volume 10, March 1984. Part of chapter 9 was published in the *Nederlands Theologisch Tijdschrift*, Spring 1987. The courtesy of the Editors of these journals, in permitting reproduction, is acknowledged.

LIST OF PARTICIPANTS

Peter Byrne BA BPhil, Lecturer in the Philosophy of Religion and a Director of the Centre of Medical Law and Ethics, King's College London

G R Dunstan MA HonDD HonLLD FSA HonMRCP, Emeritus Professor of Moral and Social Theology in the University of London

Sir Immanuel Jakobovits BA PhD HonDD HonDLitt, Chief Rabbi of Britain and the Commonwealth

E Stewart Johnson BSc MB BS PhD LRCP MRCS, Medical Director, Beecham Pharmaceuticals

John Marshall DSc MD FRCP(London) FRCP(Edinburgh) DPM, Professor of Clinical Neurology in the University of London

Elliot E Philipp MA MB FRCS FRCOG, Consulting Obstetrician and Gynaecologist, Royal Northern Hospital and Whittington Hospital (City of London Maternity Unit) London

Mary J Seller BSc PhD DSc, Reader in Developmental Genetics, The United Medical and Dental Schools of Guy's and St Thomas' Hospitals, London

A Brendan Soane BSc(Eng) PhD DIC ARSM STL, Spiritual Director of the Beda College, Rome; formerly Lecturer in Moral Theology, Allen Hall, London

1

THE STATE OF THE QUESTION
G R Dunstan

The widespread practice of *in vitro* fertilisation as a remedy for human infertility, and its attendant research on human embryos, have provoked debate all over the world, as nations try to formulate their public policies. Understanding of the fundamental cell biology and of the scientific and clinical procedures involved is not universal; indeed, both are widely misunderstood. Emotional responses cloud consideration of the moral and social issues. Pressure groups gain strength from simplified and apparently definitive presentations as they seek to hasten governments into legislation or other means of control. Religious authority is invoked. Practice in Britain, both clinical and in research, goes quietly forward under the consensual regulation of the Voluntary Licensing Authority, a body set up by the Medical Research Council and the Royal College of Obstetricians and Gynaecologists for this purpose until the government has set up an authority of its own. The British government may be ready to legislate in the near future on the basis of the report of the Warnock committee and of the responses to a consultation paper based on that report. Little time remains for the education of the public, and for a calm discussion of the questions raised. This book is written as a modest contribution to that end.

Over the past ten years a small group has been meeting at King's College London to discuss topics on medical ethics on which the traditions from which the members respectively come were thought to differ. The group produced its first book, *Consent in Medicine: Convergence and Divergence in Tradition*, in 1983.[1] Its next task was to discuss the moral status of the human embryo in a manner appropriate to the composition of the group. It comprises three medical

9

practitioners, a research scientist engaged in experimental biology, a philosopher, and three theologians working on moral questions, one of them being the Chief Rabbi of Britain and the Commonwealth. The religious traditions represented, therefore, were by design Jewish and Christian, the latter including the Anglican and the Roman Catholic. The medical and scientific members were drawn from the three religious communities. This book, like the first one, contains no more than reflections, shared in conversation, on a problem as seen in the light of personal disciplines and traditions.

The moral examination of questions like those before us – what protection is due to the human embryo and what is the extent of our liberty towards it? – requires, first, serious attention to the facts, to what is known and done; secondly, an analysis of the moral claims arising from or attending the facts, conducted out of a moral tradition; and thirdly, an estimate of moral fit, of how far the conclusions arising from the second stage commend themselves as consistent with other moral assumptions in the consciences of in-formed persons of normal competence and integrity. This pattern may be seen in the arrangement of the chapters of this book.

Chapter 2 is a simple outline of how the embryo can be seen to develop from the time when the egg or ovum of the woman and the sperm or seed of the man unite. Chapter 3 describes the ends which might be served by research of various sorts on the cleaving embryo – that is, on the cells of the zygote, morula or blastocyst in the few days of cellular fluidity before the commitment of cells to particular organic destinations initiates embryogenesis, the formation of the embryo proper. This period covers about fifteen days from fertilisation. Chapter 4 is an examination of one particular possibility, the disclosure of the sex of the nascent child, whether at the pre-embryonic, embryonic or fetal stage, with a view to choosing whether it should continue in being or be destroyed. The grounds for the choice may be medical or non-medical, and moral distinctions are drawn between them. Sex selection is not the only ethical issue attending knowledge gained from the study of the embryo. It was included here simply because it arose in our conversations, as an option now being openly discussed, and therefore one to be examined.

The second part of the book looks into the traditions. Chapter 5 is historical in method. It traces a moral tradition from the civilizations of ancient Mesopotamia through Jewish, Greek, Arabic and European cultures, and suggests a relevance to the knowledge given us and the options facing us today. Chapter 6 gives reasons why one of these options, delaying protection until the embryo has the capacity for sentience, ought not to be chosen. Chapters on Jewish Rabbinic teaching, and on contemporary Roman Catholic teaching and its attendant casuistry, follow. In chapter 9 a philosopher examines the arguments advanced and tries to discern consistency or inconsistency between them and with contemporary philosophic reasoning.

In order to set out a starting point for the examination, this chapter will now summarise a moral position which its author believes to be consistent with the understanding which enables the practitioners in research and clinical medicine to operate as they do in Britain, with historical tradition as sketched, and with such indicators as we have of a forming public opinion. Such indicators are found in the statements of professional and other organisations given in evidence to the Warnock committee, in the report of the committee, and in the opinions and practice of people who have had occasion to inform themselves of the issues at stake and, some of them, to choose and decide for themselves. It must be said at once that the statement is a personal one by its author; no other member of the group is committed to it. Later chapters in the book express reasoned dissent from it. By this means readers may be helped to decide where they themselves would stand.

Research and clinical treatment are inseparable. It is unrealistic to validate the second as the end without the first as the means. The remedies, relevant to our purpose, now offered for some forms of infertility are two: *in vitro* fertilisation followed by replacement of the embryo into the

11

uterus; and GIFT, the insertion of gametes, ova from the woman, sperm from the man, in proximity in the woman's fallopian tube in the hope that they will fertilise there. The rate of success is still very low. Both treatments are the fruit of fundamental research, that is, of observation for its own sake, followed by experimental practice. Practice included the experimental use of human embryos generated for the purpose, none of which survived to become a baby until the first successful IVF pregnancy in 1978. That birth was not achieved without extensive embryonic loss (death). So uncertain is the art at this stage of its development that only by means of more such experiment will the success rate be improved. This too will involve extensive embryonic loss (death).[2,3,4] Many of the experimental observations and procedures outlined in chapter 3, undertaken for a variety of medical reasons, will also require extensive embryonic loss (death). The question follows: are these deaths morally significant? Are we at liberty or not to bring them about for the sake of the purposes stated? Some say that we are not. Equating the moral status of the cleaving embryo with that of the human person (on the grounds that genetically it is a 'potential' person) they claim for it the protection of the Kantian rule, that a person may not be used as a means to another end, however good or beneficial to others that end may be. Support for that prohibition is evident in this book, though not necessarily for the reasons stated. What can be said on the other side?

First, that that embryonic death is not simply a wanton or indifferent addition to the death toll of nature, but is, in fact, instrumental in imposing an economy upon natural waste. In the natural order, in which man shares, there is vast wastage, inseparable from the propagation of life: frog spawn, acorns, beech mast, thistle down; millions of sperm from every man, hundreds of ova from every woman; a high percentage of embryos lost between fertilisation in natural union and implanting; to say nothing of spontaneous miscarriage. Upon this waste, medical intervention imposes an economy. If successful it provides a baby where otherwise there would be none. The genetic information stored in the cells can be read; what is thus learned can be ordered into knowledge; knowledge can be put to beneficial, life-saving use. The argument is *not* that because nature is prodigal we may be prodigal; that because so much life and potential life is lost, one more does not matter. It is the reverse. It is that nature's prodigality is turned to creative use; natural loss is lessened, albeit to a minute degree.

Secondly, it is not self-evident that the cleaving embryo has, or must be deemed to have, a moral status equivalent to that of a human person. Identity, individuality, uniqueness, does not begin at fertilisation, but long before. If any moment can be pinpointed in the ageless process of biological descent when the *possibility* of identity is laid down, by the exclusion of other possibilities, it is early in the formation of the gametes, the ova and sperm, while still separate in the bodies of the parents. At the beginning of the first meiotic division of the precursor cells, the oocytes and spermatocytes, homologous chromosome pairs (one from father and one from mother) come together and become intimately associated along their length, and in places exchange segments of genetic material. This results in a change in the versions of the component genes of each chromosome. Then, a subsequent phase of meiotic cell division randomly assigns each of the homologous chromosome pairs to the daughter cells which on maturation will form the gametes. These two processes in gametogenesis, recombination and independent assortment, ensure that the genetic constitution of each gamete is different from the next and from the parent, and are the basis of the uniqueness of the individual. The union of sperm and ovum to form the zygote does not create a new unique individual, it carries forward a process already begun. A process which does not result in identity until the time of cellular fluidity and plenipotentiality is passed, when some cells have separated to become the future embryo while others remain for placental support, and when one primitive streak has emerged on the embryonic plate as the basis for organogenesis and growth into a discrete human form.[5] The developmental process may not result in a human being at all, but in a mass of tissues like a hydatidiform mole or a chorionic carcinoma which, though compounded of human genes, is not human in any other sense of the word.

It is axiomatic in Western philosophy that there can be no personality without discrete individuality. The English common law, to look no further, does not recognise the human child as a person, that is, as a bearer of rights, until it is born alive. Neither is it sufficient to rest a claim to the status and rights of a person on the 'potential' for personality in the embryo. Roger Bacon, among the Scholastic philosophers of his day, disposed of that argument seven centuries ago.[6] The argument will not bear the weight put upon it.

To argue thus that neither the human embryo nor the human fetus is a bearer of rights is not to leave it without protection. We have duties towards it, because there is a presumption in favour of its life. The presumption is rebuttable only for grave reason. The historical chapter later in the book, chapter 5, demonstrates that in the moral, canonical and legal traditions of the West the duty of protection has always been heightened as the fetus grows towards maturity: morphology and moral claim advanced together, step by step, so that the burden of rebutting the presumption in favour of life grew ever heavier.

What, then, of the cleaving embryo, the cells in that pre-embryonic period of fluidity on the manipulation of which so much depends both in the treatment of infertility and in the search for knowledge beneficial to medicine? Even at this stage the organism is not a thing indifferent; it is precious, claiming respect, both because of its origin in human genes and because of the potential for life locked up in it. And so it is treated by embryologists who know that such respect is an essential condition of use. But it is my belief that the remedying of infertility (permitting life where otherwise there would be sheer loss) and the search for knowledge beneficial to medicine (using knowledge which otherwise would be lost) are reasons grave enough to rebut the presumption in favour of cleaving pre-embryonic life.

14

This view is not shared by everyone. Yet even some of those who reject it in principle come near to it in practice. If, out of respect for embryonic life, they insist that all fertilised ova be returned to the uterus of the mother, what, in fact, do they intend? Either that the two or three extra embryos will help in the implantation of one (as clinical experience suggests that they may), in which case they are deliberately using two or three human embryos as a means to benefit the one, in violation of their Kantian rule. Or they must hope that, in order to avoid the hazards to the mother and the babies of a high multiple pregnancy, nature will discard what scruple does not permit them to discard; and this looks like a position of moral ambiguity. The only logical position for them would seem to be to repudiate the whole treatment, leaving the infertile to seek help or consolation in other ways, and to renounce for themselves any benefits which might accrue from embryonic research.

This argument, it is repeated, is a personal one, not shared by all contributors to the book. Yet there could be claimed for it a certain moral fit; that is, consistency with what is held to be morally licit, and is practised, by informed and thinking people around us. There is a gradation in the response of grief from the loss (if noticed) of an unimplanted embryo, to an early miscarriage, to a loss later in pregnancy, to a stillbirth, to a cot death. This would correspond to that gradation in the value put upon life which is reflected in the relevant law: the indications for permissible termination of pregnancy are stricter after viability than before it, and the intentional ending of neonatal life is a crime.

The practice of post-coital contraception, where accepted, whether by means of an intra-uterine device or of hormonal compounds, rests on the assumption of equivalence with contraception rather than with abortion – for the embryo is prevented thereby from implanting in the womb – but it accepts embryonic loss. It is on this footing that an instruction approved by the Roman Catholic hierarchy in England and Wales permits the administration of the hormonal compound to a ravished woman to prevent

15

conception.[7] Genuine research studies, properly designed and conducted, to discover where the weight of moral consensus, if any, lies, are rare. One such study, however, conducted with the help of 1920 women of child-bearing age attending clinics in Edinburgh for family planning, for antenatal care, or for treatment for infertility, yielded a high response rate, ranging from 79 per cent to 96 per cent in the three groups. High percentages of respondents were in favour of IVF treatment for the infertile (94 per cent), research on the human embryo up to 14 days of growth to improve that treatment (67 per cent), and embryo research aimed at the avoidance of congenital defect (77 per cent). A majority, 70 per cent, thought that women should be permitted to donate ova for research. Religious allegiance – in a country where both Roman Catholicism and Protestantism are serious forces – was a determinant of attitude; but in no case did the majority-minority division coincide with religious profession.[8]

Here, then, is the state of the question. Treatment for infertility by IVF and GIFT is widely practised now in Britain, Europe, Israel, Australia, Canada and the USA. The attendant embryonic research is conducted on the basis of what might be called a principled pragmatism, a search for working hypotheses and solutions conducted according to recognised principles under systems of supervision or regulation differing from country to country. This chapter has sketched a rebuttable case in justification of the work. In the chapters which follow, after information necessarily given, that case will be put to the test.

References

1 G R Dunstan and M J Seller (eds) *Consent in medicine: convergence and divergence in tradition.* London, King Edward's Hospital Fund for London, 1983.
2 R G Edwards. *Conception in the human female.* London, Academic Press, 1980.
3 R G Edwards and J M Purdy (eds) *Human conception in vitro.* London, Academic Press, 1982.

4 S Fishel and E M Symonds (eds) *In vitro fertilization: past present, future*. Oxford, IRL Press, 1986.
5 M J Seller (personal communication); A McLaren. Why study early human development? *New Scientist*, 24 April 1986.
6 D C Lindberg. *Roger Bacon's philosophy of nature*. Oxford, Clarendon Press, 1983: p 11. (Quoting Bacon, *De multiplicatione specierum*, I, 1, 147–164)
7 *The Tablet*, 11 October 1986.
8 E M Alder, D T Baird, M M Lees and others. Attitudes of women of reproductive age to *in vitro* fertilization and embryo research. *Journal of Biosocial Science*, 18, 1986: pp 155– 167.

2

THE CHRONOLOGY OF HUMAN DEVELOPMENT

Mary J Seller

The process of formation of an embryo begins with gamete production. The ova and sperm are derived from the germinal epithelium of the ovary and testis, and during their formation they undergo a special form of cell division called meiosis. This has two functions. It ensures in each gamete a reduction by half of the total chromosome number, and also random recombination of the genetic elements of the cell. The significance of the latter is that the actual combination of genes carried by each gamete differs both from its parent cell and from all other cells. At *fertilisation*, a genetically unique ovum and sperm unite.

Fertilisation is not a single event which happens in a moment, but is a process. At its simplest, it involves the spermatozoon digesting a path through the membrane which surrounds the ovum, penetration of the ovum and passage through the egg cytoplasm, the formation and then fusion of the male and female pronuclei, and the coming together of the maternal and paternal sets of chromosomes.

When fertilisation has occurred, a *zygote* is formed. Cell division is then initiated and development is a continuous process. The zygote cleaves to form first two blastomeres (second day) then four (third day), and so on with increasing rapidity, the blastomeres becoming progressively smaller. Subsequently a solid ball of cells called a *morula* (fourth day) is formed. A cavity develops within the morula, transforming it into a *blastocyst* (fifth day). Implantation in the uterus begins at this stage. The outer layer of cells of the blastocyst will form the nutritive part of the conceptus – eventually the placenta – while the inner, central mass of cells will form the embryo itself and the membranes. *Conceptus* is a term which may be used for all products of conception, that is, the embryo, the placenta and membranes, at any stage of development from fertilisation to birth.

The outer cells of the conceptus proliferate and invade the uterine wall, and implantation is complete around the tenth day. The inner cell mass thickens to form a two-layered, or bilaminar, embryonic disc, which subsequently becomes trilaminar after the formation of the *primitive streak* in the midline around the fourteenth day, from which originates a third cellular component. These three cell layers are the primary germ layers which are the basic elements from which all the tissues and organs will be derived.

The trilaminar embryonic disc then elongates, proliferates rapidly, increasing markedly in size, and folds and differentiates. This is the period of *organogenesis*. The neural plate begins to form on the eighteenth day and the whole central nervous system is laid down by the twenty-sixth day. Blood vessel formation commences in the third week and a primordial heart begins to beat spasmodically and circulate blood on the twenty-second day. The arm and leg buds appear on the twenty-sixth and twenty-eighth days respectively and at the same time the primordia of the ears and eyes are laid down.

In the fifth week, the head enlarges relative to the trunk and the limbs become segmented. In the sixth week, fingers and toes become distinct and by the seventh week the embryo has a decidedly human appearance.

For the first two weeks of its existence, the growing organism is traditionally referred to as the *zygote* or *fertilised ovum* but more recently the term *pre-embryo* has been used too. For the next five or six weeks, during the period of organogenesis, it is termed an *embryo*. From the eighth week onwards, it is referred to as a *fetus*. Development thereafter essentially consists of growth and maturation of the organs and systems which have been produced during the embryonic period. Although the sex is determined at fertilisation, the two sexes cannot be distinguished externally until around twelve weeks.

19

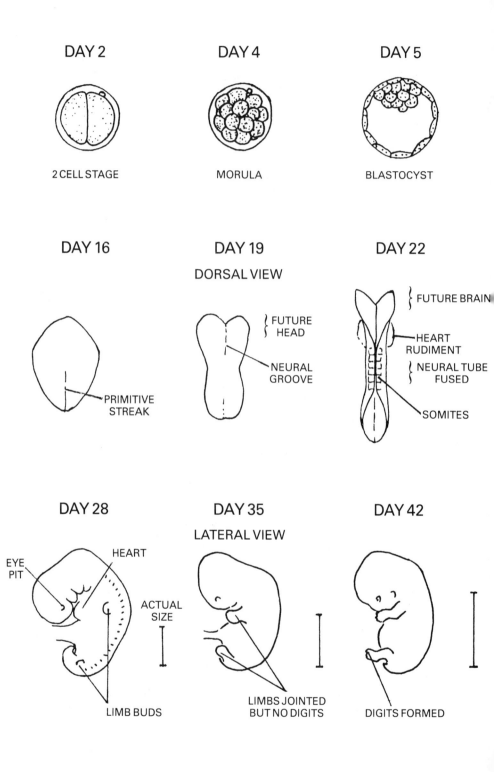

DAY 2 — 2 CELL STAGE

DAY 4 — MORULA

DAY 5 — BLASTOCYST

DAY 16 — PRIMITIVE STREAK

DAY 19 — DORSAL VIEW — FUTURE HEAD, NEURAL GROOVE

DAY 22 — FUTURE BRAIN, HEART RUDIMENT, NEURAL TUBE FUSED, SOMITES

DAY 28 — EYE PIT, HEART, ACTUAL SIZE, LIMB BUDS

DAY 35 — LATERAL VIEW — LIMBS JOINTED BUT NO DIGITS

DAY 42 — DIGITS FORMED

The *fetus* becomes an *infant* once it is outside its mother's body, whether or not the umbilical cord has been cut.

Estimation of prenatal age

The age of the embryo used in the foregoing paragraphs has been the fertilisation age, that is, calculated from the time of fertilisation. It is the true age of the embryo. Confusion can arise because pregnancies are often dated from the last menstrual period (LMP) of the mother, which occurs roughly two weeks before fertilisation. In obstetric practice, the menstrual age is almost invariably used, and the pregnancy ends approximately 40 weeks after the first day of the LMP; the fetus, however, is only 38 weeks old. Embryologists on the other hand customarily use the fertilisation age.

Twins

Twins may be dizygotic or monozygotic. Dizygotic twins (fraternal or non-identical twins) arise from the separate fertilisation of two ova and so are independent zygotes from conception. Monozygotic twins ('identical' twins) result from the fertilisation of one ovum which subsequently splits into two. Either the inner cell mass divides at the end of the first week or the beginning of the second or, less commonly, the embryonic disc splits around the twelfth day.

3

REASONS FOR WISHING TO PERFORM RESEARCH ON HUMAN EMBRYOS

Mary J Seller and Elliot Philipp

This chapter attempts solely to give a list, with some explanations, of some potential medical benefits which it is believed can be achieved by research on human embryos. It does not include investigations regarded as being simply for the pursuit of pure science. Some of the research lines mentioned are technically not yet feasible, and some might even be impossible to achieve. Further, we are not advocating that any of these lines of research *should* be pursued, or that the research should necessarily be permitted. Our intention is to be factual, and to give some idea of the sort of areas where new and useful knowledge might be obtained.

1 *Improved culture methods for IVF itself*

Present culture methods are far from foolproof, and their multiple stages of preparation give rise to the possibilities of serious errors. Ova are fertilised in one culture medium, in an incubator within a particular balance of gases (oxygen, nitrogen and carbon dioxide), then during the subsequent process of early development of the embryo, both the medium and the gas phase are altered.

However, it is not yet certain what constituents and what quantities of substances such as pyruvates are optimal for the culture of human embryos. This cannot be investigated using animals, for each species has its own individual requirements. Even the embryos of two such closely related species as the rat and mouse will not grow in exactly the same culture medium. So, finding the optimum conditions for human embryos can only be done using human embryos.

At present, not all fertilised human embryos which start

in culture actually grow successfully to be suitable for replacement in the mother. If, by experiment, another medium could be found which actually enhanced growth rather than simply supporting it, then fewer embryos would be lost during the culture process.

It is not always necessary to study the embryos themselves. Valuable information can be obtained by analysing the fluids in which embryos are cultured; but repeated changing of these fluid media could possibly endanger some embryos. The purpose of changing the fluids would be to analyse the metabolites remaining in the culture media.

2 Investigation of chromosome abnormalities

There may be reasons intrinsic to the embryo for growth failure however, namely that it has a chromosome anomaly. Another important line of research is to investigate the types of chromosome aberration, their incidence and origin, and the way they affect cell division and growth of the embryo. Studying chromosomes involves killing the embryos because the component cells have to the fixed and broken open in order to release the chromosomes.

It is already known that major chromosome anomalies occur in around 5 per cent of stillbirths and first week deaths, and in 50 per cent of recognisable miscarriages occurring in the first trimester, and it has always been thought that the incidence at conception must be very much higher.

The main types of major chromosome anomaly are:

Trisomy　　　The presence of three, instead of two, versions of a particular chromosome, giving a total of 47 chromosomes rather than 46 in each cell. For example, Down's syndrome, where chromosome number 21 is present in triplicate.

Monosomy　　Where one of a chromosome pair is missing, so that there are only 45 chromosomes in each cell.

Triploidy   Here there is an extra set of *all* chromo-
                somes in each cell, giving a total of 69.

At birth, only three of the trisomies are commonly encountered – trisomies of chromosomes 21, 18 and 13.
However, in first trimester abortions, trisomy of most other
chromosomes, and triploids, are found. This shows that,
with the exception of trisomies 21, 18 and 13, chromosome
abnormalities are largely extremely deleterious, and do not
allow the embryo to survive very long prenatally. A few
trisomies, such as those of chromosomes 1 and 17, are
hardly ever found, and the monosomies (with the exception
of X-chromosome monosomy and, very occasionally, of
chromosome 21) are never seen. It is unlikely that they do
not arise; it must rather be that they are virtually lethal.
The actual incidence of each aberration, the range of them,
how much development each will allow and how they alter
the developmental process, needs to be elucidated from
studies on pre-implantation human embryos.

Also, although many of the chromosome abnormalities
are thought to arise during the formation and maturation of
the ovum or the sperm, it is known that some must arise
during the first few divisions of the fertilised egg, and
triploidy usually arises at fertilisation. If early embryos can
be studied *in vitro*, we hope to learn how the errors arise and
how they may be prevented.

Aberrant zygotes with three pronuclei (instead of the
normal two) which can never produce a surviving child,
would seem to be particularly suitable for certain of these
studies without the need to kill embryos that could develop
into viable infants.

3   The development of techniques for genetic screening of embryos

The proposed method for producing an embryo for screening would be to split a single embryo into two separate parts
at the two or four cell stage (deliberate twinning) and allow
one part to develop further for several days *in vitro* while the

24

other was cryopreserved in liquid nitrogen at –192°C. The two embryos so produced are identical, for identical twins arise naturally in this way. The twin which is allowed to develop would, when it had reached the appropriate number of cells, be subjected to genetic testing to examine its chromosomal constitution or, using specific gene probes, to determine whether a particular mutant gene was present which would mean that the individual would have a severe genetic disease – for example, one of the haemoglobino-pathies – thalassaemia or sickle cell disease – or muscular dystrophy. The first embryo would be destroyed during this screening process, but if the tests proved that it had been normal then its twin would be recovered from the deep freeze and implanted in the mother. If, on the other hand, the tests indicated an abnormal chromosome complement or the existence of a gene for a severe disease, the second embryo too would be destroyed. Alternatively, it could be a valuable subject for further study. This technique would thus lead to the identification of embryos that are healthy, and avoid the implantation of defective embryos in hitherto infertile women, and it could also be used for couples known to be carriers of genetic disease, to allow them to implant only embryos free from the disease. These tech-niques would merely put back to an earlier stage of human development the identification of congenital disease which is now obtained from cells taken at amniocentesis, at around the sixteenth week of pregnancy, or from the study of chorionic villus biopsy specimens taken at around ten weeks. The new techniques would permit killing *in vitro* rather than, as at present, abortion *in vivo* at around either twelve weeks or twenty weeks of gestation.

4 *Gene transfer*

With further research, however, there is the possibility of 'curing' embryos found to have a mutant gene, rather than simply discarding them. This would be done by gene transfer. The correct form of the gene would be injected into the cell, or into the few cells which constitute the early embryo, and this would be incorporated in the genome (the entire genetic material, comprising all the genes, together with the intergenic DNA sequences) and would function, making good the defect. Additionally, and most importantly, this normal gene would be passed on to all the descendents of those cells, including the germ cells, making the cure permanet not only for that individual, but also for subsequent generations. Initially, while the techniques are bieng developed, it would be necessary to kill the experimental embryos.

5 Hormone production of the human embryo

This would eludicate what horomones the embryo produces to help it mature and to implant. Such research may help to lower the 25 per cent rate of spontaneous abortion which, whether the implantation has followed *in vitro* or *in vivo* fertilastion, is known to occur and is immensely distressing to women who desire to have a baby.

6 Improvement of low temperature storage techniques

At present, although embryos and sperm can be relatively easily cryopreserved, the technique for cryopreservation of ova is proving more difficult to perfect. It does seem to depend on the development of chemical substances into which the ova are placed before they are frozen. The techniques for embryo freezing are also far from perfect, many bieng damaged in the freezing and even more in the thawing process. It is highly desirous to improve storage techniques for unfertilised oocytes. This is because, for many people, it would avoid many of the ethical dilemmas which surround the freezing of whole embryos. Some of these were highlighted by the death of an American couple in a plane crash, whose two embryos were cryopreserved in Australia. To whom did these two embroys now belong? Should they have been brought to term to inherit their parents' estate? If, instead, the ova and semen of the parents had been cryopreserved, such problems would not have arisen.

7 To study certain types of male infertility

In particular, this research is needed to investigate further the fertilisation capacity of 'poor' semen, and how this can be improved. Many marriages are infertile because of low motility of spermatozoa. It is not yet known why motility is more important than numbers, and further research may help to elucidate this problem, and lead to the resolution of many cases of infertility. *In vitro* fertilisation may be the way couples so afflicted could be helped to have children of their own. Here, not only would embryos not be killed, but more might be formed from oocytes which otherwise could not be fertilised.

8 To study causes of premature labour, stillbirth, and other serious conditions of pregnancy

This research would investigate further such conditions as *abruptio placentae*, which are a common cause of premature labour and stillbirth. We do not know at all why *abruptio placentae* (bleeding behind the placenta) occurs, and it may be that there is some faulty development in the trophoblast. The trophoblast is the outer layer of the early embryo which invades the maternal uterine walls, establishes embryonic nutrition and subsequently gives rise to the placenta. Such research is vital; there were for instance 58 cases of stillbirth and neonatal death from *abruptio placentae* among the 383 perinatal deaths in the North West Thames Regional Health Authority in 1983. Although, at present, a clear path to link the condition at the end of fetal life with that at the beginning of embryonic life cannot yet be visualised, research which might be deemed purely scientific could possibly be fruitful.

9 The development of new contraceptives and abortifacients

Whether we like it or not, the fact is that well over 100,000 pregnancies are terminated yearly in the United Kingdom and the methods of termination are crude and may cause considerable damage to later fertility. Different methods of termination may be employed according to the stage of pregnancy involved. Once a pregnancy is established, and up to the end of the first trimester, the embryo is deliberately destroyed after dilatation of the cervix (neck of the womb) and suction of the contents of the womb into a glass jar. In the mid-trimester, prostaglandin induction is used. This involves the application of relatively newly discovered chemical substances into the vagina or uterus which initiate a miniature labour.

If research revealed less damaging ways of terminating the pregnancies that society allows to be terminated (because of fetal abnormalities, for example) the end result could be extra safety for the mother and a lessening of the risk to her subsequent fertility. Approved ways of fertility control would offer an alternative to these crude methods.

If research on human embryos were permitted, it may be possible to develop ways of identifying any zygotes that are at risk of developing with congenital abnormalities not associated with chromosome aberrations. We may even be able to go still further and identify the gametes that would be at risk of producing abnormal babies. This would be a large step forward because so many fetal abnormalities remain unpredictable no matter what screening tests are employed.

10 To study embryonic antigens

Cleaving embryos express unusual antigens (distinctive proteins) on their cell surfaces, many of which are similar to those found on tumours. This is one of several reasons why research on embryos may help our understanding of the mechanisms involved in cancerous growth. A large proportion of the embryos would, initially at least, be destroyed.

11 To study normal and abnormal morphogenesis

It is of cardinal importance to be able to study the normal developmental processes from the fertilised egg through to a multicellular embryo. When we know the normal mechanisms, then we have a baseline from which to study abnormal development which results in congenital malformations such as spina bifida, cleft lip and palate, and congenital heart defects, which together affect 1–2 per cent of all births. Knowledge of both normal and abnormal development is necessary if we are to reduce the total number of malformations. Such studies would involve, among other things, analysis of the initiation of gene expression and gene regulation, biochemical aspects of development, cell metabolism and cell/cell interaction.

12   Disease therapy

Embryos could provide a source of cells or tissues or organ primordia for transplantation into patients with certain diseases, as a means of therapy. It has been suggested that it might be possible, for example, to make stem cells from the embryo grow in the heart of an adult who has suffered a myocardial infarction. This would be preferable to organ transplants, and a great step forward if it could be achieved. Stems cells are undifferentiated precursor cells which have the potential both to develop into many different types of mature cells, the actual one being determined by factors such as the surrounding environment, and also to reproduce themelves. The advantage of stem cells is therefore that they are a continuously and endlessly self-renewing source of cells, which can give rise to many different cell types. Again, stem cells could also be used to replace marrow cells that have been destroyed when irradiation has been involved in the treatment of certain leukaemias. At present, bone marrow transplants seem to be the preferred method of treatment, but if such stem cell transplants could be obtained from embryos, a larger, more easily available, and antigenically less dangerous source would be available. Embryonic stem cells might also be a useful form of treatment for a number of the congenital blood disorders.

13 Would these investigations involve destruction of the embryo?

Indications as to the answer to this question have been given in the text. In summary, certain of the research possibilities mentioned above would simply involve observation of the embryo, and there would be no interference with its early development. This would mean that, at the appropriate time, the embryo could be transferred to the uterus of its mother to complete normal development to term. This would include improvement of the culture methods, elucidation of the nature of embryonic hormone production, and some, but not all, studies on the process of normal morphogenesis. Some of the research, however, might involve a risk that the embryo might be destroyed; for instance, in testing different culture conditions. On the other hand, other lines of research would necessitate the destruction of the embryo, for, by the very nature of the study, the embryo could not survive. This applies to the majority of the research possibilities mentioned: the cause and effect of chromosome abnormalities; genetic screening; treatment of genetic disease by gene transfer; causes of serious deleterious conditions of pregnancy; the development of new contraceptives; studies on embryonic antigens and normal and abnormal morphogenesis; and disease therapy.

14 Are these research possibilities feasible at present?

If research could be performed on human embryos, certain of the research lines mentioned could be pursued at once. This would include improving the culture methods, investigation of the cause and nature of chromosome abnormalities, hormone production by the embryo, investigation of male infertility, cause of *abruptio placentae*, development of new contraceptives, studies of embryonic antigens, and some studies on normal morphogenesis. There are no animal data as yet, to show whether embryonic stem cells could be used to overcome successfully the damage caused by such factors as myocardial infarction, but it is known from experiments on mice that stem cells derived from pre-implantation mouse embryos will populate the bone marrow and some other organs.

Deliberate twinning of embryos is now widely practised in farm animal breeding. In certain laboratories, genes are being inserted into mouse embryos; the success rate is not high, and some difficulty is being experienced in getting proper expression of the gene, but there is no reason why this should not soon be overcome. It would seem that it is only a small step to apply these techniques to human embryos. Gene probes for certain human diseases are now available, and the chemical sequences have been determined for some human genes. Work is progressing at an enormous pace in this field, and much effort and resources are being put into these areas. It will surely not be long before gene probes for the whole spectrum of genetic disease, and synthetic human genes, will be available. Indeed, it is likely that this chapter will be out of date by the time it is published.

Postscript

We have attempted to show the wide range of research possibilities which might be pursued on human embryos. We wish to reiterate that we are not suggesting that any of the possibilities should, or should not, be undertaken. Further, we have made no ethical comment; our purpose has been solely to be informative.

Bibliography

1 R G Edwards. The case for studying human embryos and the constituent tissues *in vitro*. In: R G Edwards and J M Purdy (eds) *Human conception in vitro*. London, Academic Press, 1982: pp 371–388.
2 R G Edwards. *Scientific and medical implications of human conception in vitro*. The Vatican, Pontificia Academia Scientiarum, 1984.

3 Embryo Research. *The Lancet*, i, 1985: pp 255–256.
4 H J Evans and A McLaren. Commentary on the Unborn children (Protection) Bill. *Nature*, 314, 1985: pp 127– 128.
5 *Human fertilization and embryology.* Submission by the Royal Society to the Department of Health and Social Security Committee of Inquiry into Human Fertilization and Embryology. London, The Royal Society, 1983.
6 A McLaren. Research on early human embryos from *in vitro* fertilization (IVF): the Warnock recommendations. *British Journal of Obstetrics and Gynaecology*, 92, 1985: pp 305–307.

4

ON SELECTING THE SEX OF THE CHILD TO BE BORN

G R Dunstan

In accepting a scientific approach to the study of the universe, we accept that knowledge is to be pursued for its own sake. This is not to say that any means whatever may be employed in the pursuit: the means must be ethical. Neither is it to say that the knowledge so gained may be put to any use whatever: there is also an ethics of the use of knowledge. In discussing research on the human embryo, the group asked itself: what use if any may properly be made of knowledge gained of the sex of the embryonic child?

It is not possible at present to contrive that any particular conception shall result in a male or a female child. There are said to be techniques or timings effective to this end, but none has yet been scientifically demonstrated. It is possible, however, to discover the sex of a conceptus at at least three points in its history. The first is at the two-cell or four-cell stage. Either the pre-embryo can be twinned artificially *in vitro* and, while the twin is preserved at low temperature, the chromosomal constitution of the other can be examined and its sex thus established; or a single cell can be taken from the pre-embryo (by embryonic biopsy), cultured and examined similarly; the pre-embryo itself will replace the cell by another.

The second point is at eight or nine weeks of growth, when chorionic villus biopsy can be performed. The chromosomal constitution of these extra-embryonic cells can be examined as before. At this stage, too, DNA analysis of the cells of a male fetus can often establish, with high but not total certainty, whether or not it bears the gene for haemophilia or Duchenne muscular dystrophy, and so will or will not be affected by the disease.

33

The third point is at sixteen to eighteen weeks, by amniocentesis, when cells taken from the amniotic fluid can be examined. At sixteen weeks also an ultrasound scan may, more often than not, show visibly the sex of the fetus.

A decision to discard the conceptus because it was not of the desired sex would involve, at the first point of intervention, not implanting the stored pre-embryo in the uterus. At the second or third points it would require the termination of the pregnancy, or, in the case of a multiple pregnancy, selective feticide, sparing the chosen while killing the unwanted. Termination of pregnancy is regarded with distaste by many; by some with abhorrence. It is an operative procedure which involves risk to the mother. Sex selection at the pre-embryo stage involves virtually no risk, and is relatively easy.

A clinical justification for such intervention to eliminate a conceptus of a particular sex is advanced for families at risk from the serious X-linked disorders such as haemophilia or Duchenne muscular dystrophy, when specific tests show that the deleterious gene is present in the conceptus. When this occurs, a female child would carry the condition but not the manifestation of it; a male child could be affected. DNA studies can now determine whether the male child is affected or not. To avoid the risk of the disease occurring in this generation, a male pre-embryo or fetus would be destroyed. To avoid the risk of transmitting the gene to a subsequent generation, the female would be destroyed. To accept a trouble-free life in this generation without regard to the next, the female would be preserved. (It is a further question, not pursued here, whether she could or should then be sterilised later in life to avoid the possible transmission of the gene.)

That clinical justification would be rejected by those who would apply to nascent human life at any stage – pre-embryo, embryo, fetus – the absolute protection which, they claim, is due to 'innocent' human life. For some of these that claim is warranted and fortified by the will of God and, for some again, by an alleged unbroken tradition in the Church. Leaving aside the theological claim and the appeal to tradition, it may be observed that the word 'innocent' is not without moral ambiguity. In the context of the protection due to human life it is not the equivalent of morally or legally blameless. It means causing or threatening no harm. (The old adage may be recalled, *primum non nocere*: first of all, to do no harm.) An enemy soldier in time of war is a legitimate target for attack while he threatens harm, without consideration for his moral culpability for the war or for anything else; as soon as he is disabled or disarmed and so incapable of threatening harm, he is entitled to the protection due to innocent life.

If this casuistry be now applied to nascent human life, it would justify its termination if the fetus threatened serious harm to the mother, but for no other indication – unless the carrying of a recessive deleterious gene were held to be a serious threat to a child in a future generation. To terminate on the grounds that, if the fetus went to term and were born, the child would suffer grave handicap, must rest on the supposition that it were better not to live at all than to live with handicap of varying degree of severity. The child-to-be would be killed in its own assumed interest. A justification of this sort is much disputed. Its acceptance or rejection – by prospective parents, for example, receiving genetic counselling – would require consideration of the statistical probability or diagnostic certainty of the congenital factor, of the predicted or estimated degree of handicap, and an estimate of the parents' capacity to care for and to rear a child so afflicted in a way which would make the affliction tolerable. It would require finally, under the present British law, the parents' own judgment and choice whether to ask for termination or not.

These considerations will be recognised as normal to the debate on therapeutic abortion, now applied to the special case of a pre-embryo, embryo or fetus known to carry an X-linked deleterious gene.

A further question is asked: should potential parents be allowed the liberty to establish or continue a pregnancy only if the sex diagnosed matched their present wish? Or, to put the question another way: should parents be allowed

35

the liberty to discard or abort if the sex diagnosed were not that of the son or daughter they would wish for? Genetic clinics are being asked increasingly (though the request is seldom granted) for sex determination simply for the sake of having a child of the sex preferred. There is no question here of genetic handicap.

Those who claim absolute protection for nascent life would be on surer ground here. They could be fortified by a theological doctrine of providence; a general providence, perhaps, a belief that a wise and loving God had so ordained the procreative process (for mankind as for a wide compass of the biological order) as to produce an overall balance of the sexes conducive to His good purpose for His creation, and that man must not presume wantonly (that is, for his mere convenience or pleasure) to interfere with it. Or it might be a particular providence, that in the infinite and eternal mind of God there is a vocation, a purpose, for every human soul and that sexuality, being a man or a woman, is so much a part of personality that to interfere at this point would frustrate that purpose and so be impious. The essence of humanity is a capacity for relationship, with other human, rational and companionable selves, and with the all-loving God in whose image man is made. These are propositions of faith, binding on those who profess them. To seek to overturn them by rational argument would be futile. To pursue the attempt would also be lacking in respect for conscientious conviction, personal faith and liberty; and this respect theology and ethics combine to uphold.

Against this argument would be stated the contemporary individualist libertarian claim: if we want a girl (or a boy) and can have one, why should we not? It is *our* child, whom *we* shall bring up, sharing *our* life; what right (*sic*) have other people to impose their views on us? Some would go further, and invest their claim to sovereign procreational liberty with the status of a 'right' – 'we have *a right* to the child of our choice' without stopping to ask on what that 'right' is founded. To those who advance such a claim it is self-authenticating.

But not to others. Those two parents are members of a wider society, as their child will be in its turn. That society is tolerant of personal claims: on some, indeed, it confers the status of rights; on others, of mere liberties. But it confers those rights and recognises those liberties only in relation to its own common interest. On no human being does it confer the status of property, of being possessable – the unexpressed fantasy implicit in the notion of 'choosing a child of our own'. The concept of humanity underlying this discussion presupposes man as a social being and his life to be in interplay between personal good, personal fulfilment, and social good, social fulfilment. And the claim to bear only a child of chosen sex may conflict with the social good, and therefore could not be admissible.

The strength of that objection varies with different societies. In a society like those of western Europe, where boys and girls are valued roughly equally, the exercise of choice, even if (which is doubtful) it were widely exercised, would probably not seriously threaten the rough balance of the sex ratio which is achieved naturally. (Families with an inbuilt occupational or dynastic bias in favour of sons, like the descent of titles of honour through male heirs, are statistically rare.) Successful interventions in the fields of nutrition, medicine and public health, and a prolonged period without decimating wars, do in fact change the sex ratio by reducing mortality among infant and young males, so leaving undiminished the slight imbalance of males over females at birth. But that is a secondary consequence of public measures taken on other grounds, not the direct consequence of personal choices. In societies, however, in which males are strongly favoured over females, for reasons of religion or culture or for assumed greater security against poverty and destitution in old age, the exercise of choice in the sex of children would seriously unbalance the sex ratio and hence, in a very short time, the population structure. The social and demographic consequences of males heavily outnumbering females would be serious indeed. (Modern China, implementing a policy of one child per family, may well incur these consequences, particularly if, as is alleged,

37

in areas remote from supervision girl babies may be sacrificed in order that the one permitted child shall be a boy.)

A second argument against the liberty of choice is
advanced even for societies where the threat of sexual
imbalance is not serious. It concerns the real fulfilment or
happiness or interest of the couple concerned which may
not be well served by indulgence of the passing whim which
they may feel. There are limits to the choices which people
should be asked to make because there are limits to their
capacity consciously to make them. The dogma of 'informed consent', for instance, in medical matters, if carried
to an extreme, may lay burdens of decision on patients
which they are not competent to carry. Or the insistence of
some paediatricians on leaving to parents the decision over
the management of a severely handicapped newly born
child – a decision which may result in its early death or in
its continuing a severely crippled life – may impose improper
psychological strain at the time of decision and a legacy of
guilt thereafter. There is genuine freedom in abandonment,
as there is in choice. A couple which recognises their inter-
dependence in both the biological and the social orders,
may find their happiness more in acceptance of what the
procreative lottery gives them, a boy or a girl, than in
choosing one or the other. To stand on such an argument,
and to base a policy upon it, may incur the slogan charge of
paternalism. Yet a wise society should and does develop its
conventions and rules normally to coincide with the grain
of human nature, with the promoting of what is commonly
accepted to be the happier way, judging these, not by cults
or enthusiasms which excite the popular imagination for a
time and then fade away, but by what appears to be the
common experience in long continuance of time.

At the heart of the question stands the infinite value put
upon human life. By imputing inferior value to one sex or
the other that value is lessened, trivialised. The calculation
of personal preference for a child of one sex or the other
diminishes the awe in which we stand before both. And
stand in awe we should.

38

5

THE HUMAN EMBRYO IN THE WESTERN MORAL TRADITION

G R Dunstan

There are compelling reasons, theological, philosophical and practical, why moralists should affirm the sacredness of human life. The task is the more urgent when every day brings news of assassinations, murder by terrorists, secret police and soldiery under the command of despotic governments; of wars, invasions and insurrections; of widespread death from starvation; of torture and unjust imprisonment as instruments of political oppression. The memory of inhumane 'experiments' imposed by medical scientists under the Nazi and other régimes is still painful, and dictates continual vigilance. The spread of clinically induced abortions throughout the technically-advanced countries of the world, as social expedients well beyond therapeutic necessity, calls into question the dedication of the medical profession as the servant and protector of life. It is to be expected, therefore, that those who feel most strongly that the sacredness of human life is under new threat should stake their claim at the highest conceivable point; and, indeed, that despairing of any 'half-way house' or defensible intermediate point, should claim 'absolute' protection for the human embryo from the moment 'when life begins'. Unless a stand is made, no life is safe; whatever experiment or disposal is thought to be expedient will somehow be justified.

Desperate situations evoke desperate remedies; but not always the right remedies. Upon examination the absolutist argument proves to offer less security than is claimed for it. First, its empirical base is not secure. The absolutists' claim that life begins 'at the moment of conception' is disputed by biologists competent to judge. Their contention is that 'life' exists independently in sperm and egg-cell before fertilisation. But not all products of conception from human gametes are recognisably human, and given the range of convolutions possible during the early stages of cell division, conception does *not* invariably determine the identity of the human person. These facts cannot be over-thrown by mere dogmatic assertion and reassertion to the contrary. One of the three bodies representing the Roman Catholic community which gave evidence to the Warnock committee, the Social Welfare Commission of the Catholic Bishops' Conference (England and Wales), has conceded the point in so far as it professes agnosticism as to when precisely life begins, though it would 'err on the side of caution' in giving the embryo the benefit of the doubt and in claiming protection for it from 'the beginning' – when-ever that is.[1] Responsible Roman Catholic moralists now argue similarly.[2,3]

Secondly, it must be replied that in neither Christian morality, Jewish morality, the Arab and Islamic traditions nor English law is human life given absolute protection at any stage. It enjoys a very high presumption in its favour, a presumption rebuttable only in terms recognised by morality and law. Morality and law may not always coincide on the definition of those terms; but that they exist there is no dispute. To claim an 'absolute' right to life for the embryo or fetus would be morally odd: the claim is inconsistent with other accepted moral claims.

Thirdly, the claim to absolute protection for the human embryo 'from the beginning' is a novelty in the western, Christian and specifically Roman Catholic moral tradi-tions. It is virtually a creation of the later nineteenth century, a little over a century ago; and that is a novelty indeed as traditions go. To recall that tradition is the purpose of this chapter.

The tradition is, in fact, well documented in authentic Roman Catholic scholarship. Many of the evidences for it are set out in the *Dictionnaire de Théologie Catholique*[4] and the *Dictionnaire de Droit Canonique*[5]; others become evident

40

when the language of the tradition is recognised and given its contextual significance. The main evidences are found in the philosophical discussion of animation – the relation of the soul to the human person – and in the moral and legal sanctions for abortion. The purpose of this chapter, however, is not to re-open the philosophical speculations upon animation nor to discuss sanctions for abortion; it is simply to recall the fact of the tradition and of its persistence in English law and Catholic moral theology and canonical jurisprudence. The philosophical notion of animation did not create the tradition – it existed before Aristotle formulated the theory; and its persistence long after the philosophical theory had lost its appeal and its point suggested that it ministered satisfactorily to a perennial human need. The need is to have some practical working rule by which to adjust conflicting and legitimate human claims in areas of moral judgment where absolutes are unattainable.

We may pick up the tradition among the civilisations of the Levant out of which some of the laws of the Old Testament were shaped. The Babylonian Code of Hammurabi prescribed compensation due for striking a woman so as to cause her to lose the child of her womb. The damages were graded according to her status: ten shekels, or five, or two, according to whether she were the daughter of a noble or a freeman, a commoner or a villein, or a slave respectively. And if she also died, the damages were similarly graded: the life of the assailant's daughter for the first category; diminishing payments for the second and third.[6,7] The Hebrew law of *Exodus* 21:22f similarly relates the compensation to the hurt to the woman, though without explicit social grading:

> And if men strive together, and hurt a woman with child, so that her fruit depart, and yet no mischief follow; he shall be surely fined, according as the woman's husband shall lay upon him; and he shall pay as the judges determine. But if any mischief follow, then thou shalt give life for life . . .

41

The Assyrian laws were similar, punishing the assault severely as an invasion of the husband's property. The Hittites, however, grounded their damages, not on the social status of the mother or on the hurt done to her, but on the gestational age of the fetus: ten shekels of silver for a ten months fetus, five shekels if the pregnancy were in its fifth month.[8]

There follows a highly significant departure. When the Hebrew text of *Exodus* was translated into Greek in the Septuagint version (LXX) in the third century BC, the Hittite principle, of relating the penalty to gestational age, was substituted for the other: compensation was payable if the fetus is *me exeikonismenon* – not yet so formed as to be a copy or portrayal of the human form; if it were *exeikonismenon*, then life was to be given for life. The LXX was followed in the Old Latin versions, evidenced before the end of the second century AD – as it was closely paralleled by the Samaritan and Karaite versions.[9] The Septuagint was the version most commonly used by the early Christian fathers (as well as by the New Testament writers); and the language of the Old Latin versions became the language of the moral tradition of the west: *Si . . . exierit infans nondum formatus . . . ; si autem formatus fuerit . . .* Thomas of Chobham, for instance, in his representative manual for confessors, *Summa Confessorum*, AD 1216, distinguishes the degrees of culpability in feticide:

> For in this matter it is written in the law of Moses 'If anyone should strike a pregnant woman and she should miscarry, if the fetus has been formed let him give life for life; if, however, it is unformed, let him be amerced in money'. From this it is clear that it is a much graver sin to dislodge a formed fetus than an unformed one.[10]

St Jerome's translation of the Hebrew text into the Latin of the Vulgate, towards the end of the fourth century, did not overthrow the Septuagint tradition. It is the distinction drawn in the LXX and Old Latin versions which appears throughout the canonical legislation of the West. It did so, we may surmise, because the moral rule was consistent both

42

with current philosophical perceptions of the relation of soul and body, and with the physiology developed in Hippocratic and Galenic medicine.

The Hippocratic *corpus* records a variety of observations on fetal growth. For 'formation' estimates are for 35 or 40 or 50 days; for the first distinguishing of limbs, about 40 days; for movement, 70, 80, 90 or 100 days; for completion to birth, from 210 to 300 days.[11] Philosophical speculation was related to these observations. In Aristotle's usage, the 'soul' (*psyche*) or animating principle (from the Latin, *anima*) was that which gave to a substance or organism its characteristic form. So, in a passage in *On the Generation of Animals*, Aristotle attributed to the earliest embryo a vegetative existence animated or informed by a 'nutritive' soul; to the later embryo, resembling a little animal, a 'sensitive' soul; to the formed fetus, recognisably human, a 'rational' or 'intellectual' soul, encapsulating not replacing the other two.[12,13] It remains to add that since the anatomy of the male distinguished its humanity by about 40 days, while doubt remained about the female until 90 days[14], these were the limits within which, in the later moral tradition, a fetus was held to be *formatus et animatus* and so indisputably human. And whereas the deliberate destruction of nascent human life at any stage was held to be a sin – like *coitus interruptus* – the penalties were graded on the basis of that distinction.

Before the *catena* of evidences is displayed, notice must be taken of two apparent dissentients from the tradition. The first was Tertullian, the North African lawyer who wrote vigorously in defence of Christianity against charges of human sacrifice, secret homicide, infanticide and other enormities. He wrote:

> For us, indeed, homicide having been forbidden once and for all, it is not lawful to destroy what is conceived in the womb even while the blood is being drawn into a humar being. To deny birth is to hasten homicide; for it makes no difference whether you snatch away the soul after birth or destroy it while coming to birth. Even the

man who is yet to be is a man, just as every fruit is already present in seed. (Apologia, 9.8).

Although Tertullian does not specify any stage of gestation, it would appear from his use of the words *dum adhuc sanguis in hominem delibatur* that his prohibition would apply early as well as late; though it is to be observed that Tertullian was by no means accounted orthodox in other of his controversial opinions, particularly in his 'transducianism' or peculiar belief that the soul (*anima*) derived from the parental seed, a belief that would give added importance to the early embryo.

A stronger witness, not tainted by heterodoxy, is St Basil (circa 330–379), Bishop of Caesarea, who expressly repudiates this tradition:

> A woman who deliberately destroys a fetus is answerable for murder. And any fine distinction as to its being completely formed or unformed (*ekmemorphomenou kai anexeikonistou*) is not admissible among us. (*Ep* clxxxviii, *Ad Amphilochium* II)

Whether or not St Basil's judgment persisted in the Greek churches, the present writer does not know, for he has not pursued the question.

The first witness against St Basil, however, and in the long chain of evidence in the West, is Basil's own brother, St Gregory of Nyssa (circa 330–395). For him, Basil's 'fine distinction' between unformed embryo and formed, animated fetus is sufficiently accepted as to be used as a premise in a theological argument:

> For just as it would not be possible to style the unformed embryo a human being, but only a potential one – assuming that it is completed so as to come forth to human birth, while so long as it is in this unformed state it is something other than a human being – so our reason cannot recognize as a Christian one who has failed to receive, with regard to the entire mystery, the genuine form of our religion. (*Adversus Macedonianos*)

44

This distinction persisted throughout the centuries in the determination of what is or is not homicide, and in the determination of canonical penances for causing a miscarriage.

First, St Augustine of Hippo (354–430):

> If what is brought forth is unformed (*informe*) but at this stage some sort of living, shapeless thing (*informiter*), then the law of homicide would not apply, for it could not be said that there was a living soul in that body, for it lacks all sense, if it be such as is not yet formed (*nondum formata*) and therefore not yet endowed with its senses. (*Quaestionum in Hept*, I II n 80)

The Celtic Penitentials were as severe as they were precise in their penal tariffs. The Bigotian canons, and the *Canones Hibernenses* (circa 665) precribes three and a half years on bread and water respectively for the destruction of 'the liquid matter of the infant in the womb' (the usual term in Galenic anatomy for the forming embryo); but fourteen and seven and a half years respectively for the destruction of 'flesh and soul' (*carnis et animae*). The Old Irish Canons had three stages: 'after it has become established in the womb (three and a half years); 'if the flesh has formed' (seven years); and 'if the soul has entered it' (fourteen years).[15]

The canon law and moral discipline of the Catholic West did not develop on Celtic lines; but the basic distinction remained entrenched. Pope Innocent III, that great legislator, issued in 1211 a canon (5.20) *De homicidio voluntario vel casuali*, determining for what offence a priest incurred 'irregularity', that is, was suspended from his priestly ministrations. So, if he had been a party to a miscarriage:

> If the conceptus is not yet quickened (*vivificatus*) he may minister; otherwise, he must abstain from the service of the altar.

The point was taken up by Raymond de Penafort (1185–1275), a major canonist, in words which influenced incidentally the formation of the English common law. He is answering the question, If someone strikes a pregnant woman or gives her poison (or she herself takes it) so that she miscarries or does not conceive, should he be adjudged a homicide or irregular? He answers:

> If the fetus (*puerperium*) is already formed or animated (*formatum sive animatum*) that is truly homicide if because of that blow or potion the woman miscarries, for he has killed a man. If however it is not yet animated, it is not said to be homicide so far as concerns irregularity, but it is accounted homicide in regard to penance. (*Summa de casibus poenitentiae*, II 1 *De homicidio*)

Henry of Bracton, Raymond's contemporary, writing on the subject in his treatise *On the Laws and Customs of England*, used words so close to Raymond's as to suggest either quotation from Raymond or use of a common source.[16] His subject is the division of the crime of homicide:

> Should anyone strike a pregnant woman or give her poison on account of which she miscarries, if the fetus is already formed and animated, and especially if animated, he commits homicide.

And among his exceptions to the criteria for the recognition of legal personality at birth:

> Item, if the issue is not formed as a human being (*non formatus ut homo*) but as a monster. (*De Legibus et Consuetudinibus Anglie*, F 120 437)

The canon law and the English common law were thus, for their respective purposes, in step. Inevitably the philosophical notion of animation became identified with the subjective experience of quickening; so quickening became a determining point for various purposes in the common law. Blackstone wrote in his *Commentaries* (fourth edition 1770) that 'Life begins in contemplation of law as soon as an infant is able to stir in the mother's womb'; and 'to be saved from the gallows a woman must be quick with child – for barely with child, unless he be alive in the womb, is not sufficient.' (i 129; iv 388). And so the law operated: in July

1387 at the Winchester assize, a gentlewoman was condemned to death for consenting and aiding in the murder of
her husband by his chaplain, but her execution was respited
because of her pregnancy; the judgment was confirmed in
the King's Bench after Easter and she was executed on 17
April 1388.[17]

Meanwhile the moral tradition continued without such
crudities and finds expression in other great figures of the
thirteenth century, notably Roger Bacon, Albertus Magnus,
St Thomas Aquinas and Dante. St Thomas is answering
the question: Is he who kills another by accident guilty of
homicide? Referring to the law of *Exodus* 21:22–3, he
writes:

> He who strikes a pregnant woman by that act puts
> himself in the wrong, so that if death should result either
> for the woman or for the animated fetus (*puerperii
> animati*) he cannot escape the crime of homicide, par-
> ticularly since it is so obvious that death may result from
> such a blow. (*Summa Theologiae*, 2a2ae 64.8)

It is indicative of how far the Aristotelian tradition is
forgotten even among such scholars as the Dominican
editors of the new Blackfriars edition of the *Summa*, that
the word *animati* is overlooked in Marcus Lefébure's translation in volume 38 of that edition. Yet St Thomas meant
what he wrote: when he writes of the relation of the soul to
embryonic growth he quotes Aristotle precisely.

> In the natural way of generation the progression is from
> the imperfect to the perfect. Hence, just as in the gen-
> eration of man first comes a living thing, then the animal,
> and finally man, so things which merely live, like plants,
> commonly exist for the sake of animals, and animals for
> the sake of men. (*Summa Theologiae*, 2a2ae 64.1)

> . . . this prime factor in intellectual activity, whether we
> call it mind or intellectual soul (*anima intellectiva*), is the
> formative principle of the body. And this is how Ari-
> stotle proves it in the *De Anima*. (*Summa Theologiae*, 1a
> 76.1)

47

... everything has its species determined by its formative principle. So we are left with this, that the intellective principle is the formative principle determining man as a species. (*Summa Theologiae*, 1a 76.1).

Besides, Aristotle says that the embryo is an animal before it is a man ... So the intellectual soul is not the same as the sensitive soul in man, but presupposes it as the matter it energizes. (*Summa Theologiae*, 1a 76.3)

... the conception of a male is not completed (*non perficitur*) until about the fortieth day, as Aristotle says in the 9th *de animalibus*; that of a female not until about the ninetieth day. (*Commentarium in Sententiis* Lib III; dist III; quest 5; art 2)

It was to these passages in St Thomas, and so to Aristotle behind him, that Catholic moralists were appealing down to the end of the nineteenth century.

Dante, meanwhile, embodied the same doctrine in his poetry. Statius, climbing with Dante to the seventh cornice of the mount of Purgatory, explains the generation of the embryo from the mingling of paternal seed with maternal blood, and its passing through the vegetable and animal stages to become a fetus:

> Apri a la verità che viene il petto;
> e sappi che si tosto come al feto
> l'articular del cerebro è perfetto,
> lo motor primo a lui si volge lieto
> sopra tanta arte di natura, e spira
> spirito novo di virtù repleto,
> che ciò trova attivo quivi tira
> in sua sustanzia, e fassi un'alma sola,
> che vive e sente, e sè in sè rigira.
> (*Purgatorio*, Cant 25; 67–75)

> Open thy heart now and the truth expect;
> and know that to the *foetus*, once the brain
> is shaped there in each last minute respect,
> the primal Mover turns himself, full fain

of nature's masterpiece, a work so fair,
and inbreathes a new spirit, which draws amain,
replete with power, all it finds active there
into its substance and becomes but one
quick, sentient soul, of its own self aware.
(Translation by Bickersteth[18])

It is to be noted that sentience and awareness, which Dante attributes to the fetus into which, now that it is formed enough to receive it, God has inbreathed the soul, are also the capacities which some modern embryologists cite as determining the point at which the fetus becomes an ethical *persona*, that is, a being with its own claims and interests which investigators and researchers must not violate.[19,20] These depend, of course, on the stage of development of the nervous system, at about the sixth week of gestation.

What Statius described was standard medieval teaching: three stages of ensoulment, the process being completed with the full form of the body at about forty days. It appears in an early thirteenth century compilation, possibly made in Gloucester Abbey.[21] It was elaborated by the celebrated Tudor surgeon, Thomas Vicary, in his treatise *The Anatomie of the Bodie of Man*, first published in 1548, and republished and revised by his colleagues at St Bartholomew's Hospital in 1577.[22] He cites as his authorities 'the noble Philosophers, as Galen, Auicen (Avicenna) and Bartholomeus', but his material is recognisably Aristotelian also; and certainly it would hardly survive the Vesalian revolution in anatomy. He describes the development of the 'Embruon' into the 'Fettus' in four stages, of which

> The fourth and laste, as when al other members be perfectly shapen, then it receyeth the soule wyth life and breath; and then it beginneth to moue it-selfe alone. . . . So is there xlvj dayes from the day of conception vnto the day of ful perfection and receyuing of the soule, as God best knoweth.

The anatomy and the philosophical speculation are alike transitory; both passed with the coming of new knowledge and new ways of thinking, methods of forming ideas. And as such we treat them – as transitory. But they were important to us as carriers of a moral tradition; they provided the forms in which moral judgments were expressed and degrees of culpability were decided. Twenty years or so after Vicary's death Pope Sixtus V, in the bull *Effraenatum* of 29 October 1588, summarily abolished the tradition which measured culpability with the development of the fetus, whether it were *formatus* and *animatus* or still *informis* and *inanimatus*:

> By this our constitution, to be valid in perpetuity, we decree and ordain that all henceforth who by themselves or by the hand of any intermediary procure the abortion or ejection of an immature fetus, whether animate or inanimate, formed or unformed, ... and also the pregnant women themselves who knowingly do the same, shall incur, by the very act (*eo ipso*) the penalties set forth and inflicted by divine as well as human law against actual murderers (*veros homicidas*).

Included in the same condemnation is the giving of potions to induce sterility or to prevent conception. And the penalty was excommunication *ipso facto* without the possibility of absolution even at the point of death. In so doing he attempted to realign the canon law with the Vulgate translation of *Exodus* 21:22f; for the Council of Trent had decreed that this translation alone should be treated as authentic.

Nevertheless, moralists and canonists alike received the bull with consternation. The next pope, Gregory XIV, was quick to modify it. In the bull *Sedes Apostolica*, 31 May 1591, he permitted local Ordinaries to relax the excommunication; and added:

> The penalties for procuring the abortion of an inanimate fetus or for administering or taking potions to cause women to be sterile we revoke just as if that constitution so far as it concerns these things had never been issued.

The moralists were thereby freed to resume their casuistry. Cornelius a Lapide SJ, in his *Commentary on the Pentateuch*,

1617, expounded the Hebrew and the Greek variants in *Exodus* 21:22f, quoting both. He equates the guilt incurred by causing the death of the fetus with that of causing the death of the mother if the fetus is *iam animatus*. He interprets the Greek, *exeikonismenon*, as *virunculus*, *uti flandrice puerum vocamus manneken*, 'a little man, called in Flemish a manneken'

> that is, if the child is shaped or formed (*effigiatus vel efformatus*), as if to say: If the child has its members perfect, so that it is fully shaped, as if it were what one might call a tiny man (*quasi parvus quidam vir*) or *virunculus*; then he who by his blow causes the pregnant woman to miscarry shall give life for life. . . . And from these words of the Septuagint it is clear that the fetus is animated at the time when it is formed (*simul atque formatus est, animari*); for on that account he who has caused it to miscarry is accounted and punished as one who commits homicide. And the Doctors teach the same.

John de Lugo SJ, a little later, in *Responsa Moralia* (1651), applying the principle of secondary or double effect when a medicine given to a mother for her good causes her to miscarry, writes:

> If the medicine has use for the life of the mother but as an unintended consequence causes her to miscarry, then, so be that the fetus is not animated, the use is licit.

A century later St Alphonsus Liguori, the most celebrated pastor and writer on moral and spiritual theology of his time, who was canonised in 1839, and whom Pius IX was to declare a Doctor of the Church in 1871, expounded the casuistry of the question in his *Theologia Moralis* (2 volumes, 1753 and 1755). His treatment of it, however, will be most easily studied in the text of an editor who had to accommodate his teaching to the intervention of Pius IX in 1869.

By the mid-nineteenth century advances in medicine were making abortion by direct assault upon the fetus both possible and safer, supplanting the indirect methods employed hitherto. The incidence of abortion therefore rose.

The rise was seen as a moral threat calling for drastic remedy. Pius IX, therefore, in the bull *Apostolicae Sedis* of 12 October 1869, declared excommunicate all who procured abortion, without distinction either as to the method, direct or indirect, intentional or involuntary, or as to the gestational age of the fetus, whether it were formed or unformed, animate or inanimate. This sentence is repeated in the most recent edition of the *Codex Iuris Canonici*, 1983, Lib VI, Tit VI, can 1398.

The effect of Pius IX's bull is seen in an edition of Liguori's *Theologia Moralis* published by J Aertnys, with an *imprimatur*, in 1896. In Lib III, Tract V, cap IV, art II he sets out, first the principles, then the questions arising, concerning abortion.

> 190   *Principles* 1:   It is never lawful *directly* to procure an abortion, even though the fetus may be supposed to be still inanimate. And for this reason: that, if the fetus is animate, homicide properly so called is committed, and that the more heinous because very often the soul is at the same time deprived of eternal life; if it is not yet animate, it is nevertheless alive (*vivus*), and is unjustly prevented from becoming a man, and this is, so to speak (*velut*) anticipated homicide; and in consequence this is more unnatural (*contra naturam*) than pollution . . .

The second Principle applies 'double effect' to permit *indirect* abortion resulting from a remedy necessarily administered to a pregnant woman to obviate a threat to her life – provided that no other remedy were available, and that the fetus were not deprived of a reasonable hope of baptism. Then come the Questions.

> 192   *Question 1:*   At what time is the fetus informed with a rational soul?
> *Response:* That it is infused once the body is sufficiently formed, at the thirtieth or fortieth day in fact, is certain, and so many hold. It is, however, more probable, and today commonly accepted, that it is infused at the very moment of conception; the rational soul, indeed, is the form which fashions the organic body (*forma plasmativa*

corporis organici) or forms the human organism. This is confirmed by the feast of the Immaculate Conception of the Blessed Virgin Mary. The contrary opinion holds that the body before the organs are formed is not apt to receive the rational soul; but this is a gratuitous claim, and, moreover, it proves too much, for the body does not exist as an instrument apt for rational operations except after birth.

Aristotle, whom the Schoolmen followed, taught that the male fetus was informed with a rational soul on the fortieth day, the female on the eightieth; and this opinion the external forum of the Church follows (*sequitur*) so far as ecclesiastical penances are to be incurred, with one exception. That wide disparity between the animation of male and female rests on no solid foundation.

Question 9: Whether those who procure an abortion incur the penalties when there is doubt whether the fetus is or is not animate?
Response 1: So far as excommunication is concerned, the answer must be Yes; for Pius IX makes no distinction between the animate and the inanimate fetus.

2: As for the other penalties, the answer should be more truly No (*verius negandum*): (a) because irregularity is not to be admitted except in cases set down in law; and the Canons speak only of cases which clearly constitute *de facto* homicide; and in this case, where there is doubt whether the fetus is animate, there is doubt also about the fact of homicide; (b) because in cases of doubt the fact may not be presumed but must be proved; (c) because in the matter of penances, the more favourable interpretation is to be followed. Hence when there is doubt whether the aborted fetus is masculine or feminine, the penalties are not incurred before the eightieth day. (Aertnys, 1896)

The process of adaptation of the moral tradition in this text is clear. Aertnys, a Redemptorist Father, expounds as closely as he may the teaching of the founder of his Order, Liguori, but qualifies it where necessary, as he was bound, by rulings of the Papacy and the Holy Office promulgated since Liguori wrote, as well as by authoritative theological opinions. Hence the reliance, not only on Pius IX's *Apostolicae Sedis*, but also on his bull of 1854 in which he established as an article of the Catholic faith the dogma of the Immaculate Conception of the Blessed Virgin Mary. Running through the cases discussed (and more are omitted here than are cited) runs Liguori's 'equiprobabilism', his teaching that when there is doubt whether substantive law exists, the laxer course is to be followed. And it was for this virtue, perhaps, that he was described by Pius IX as 'the helmsman of the safest course between laxism and rigorism' (*laxismi et rigorismi tutissimus depulsor*) and by Leo XIII as 'the most prudent of guides for directors of souls' (*animarum moderatorum prudentissimus dux*).

Conclusion

This chapter has traced one route, that of Christian philosophy, Catholic moral theology and canon law, and the English common law, by which a moral tradition passed from the civilisations of Mesopotamia through the Greeks and the Western Church into modern times. It passed by another route also. Greek philosophy and science travelled eastwards as well as westwards: some from Alexandria, some from Constantinople with the exiled Nestorian Christians into Persia and beyond. The Greek authors were translated into Syriac and Arabic. They were commented on; enriched with the lore of India and the East; worked into a coherent whole by the physician-philosophers of the ninth and tenth centuries, notably Rhazes, Beruni, Avicenna, and then Averroes; absorbed into the religion and practice of Islam; and taken by Maimonides into Rabbinic Judaism. When translated into Latin in the eleventh and twelfth centuries, in the Moorish cities of Spain and southern Italy, they reinforced what was known in the West of Aristotle and the Greeks, so engendering a new surge of philosphy and science in Albertus Magnus, Robert Grosseteste, St Thomas Aquinas and Dante. Even Chaucer's

Doctour of Phisik had the great Arabs on his bookshelf. And the Arabs maintained the same moral tradition, of grading status and protection with embryonic growth. Avicenna stated the matter simply: 'a soul comes into existence whenever a body suitable for it comes into existence'. Islamic law graded the reparation due for causing a miscarriage as the Septuagint had; though some hadith traditions in Islam permitted abortion up to a date far later than anything countenanced in the Christian West. The morally significant fact stands out: that the modern biological understanding of conception as a process not yielding individual identity until after 14 or 15 days is matched by a moral tradition of great antiquity and ubiquity which graded status and protection step by step with emerging recognisable human form. And whatever else has varied in our confused moral tradition, it has been consistent in affirming that, without discrete individuality, there can be no moral or legal personality. What Boethius (circa AD 480–524) wrote of the person, that it is 'an individual partaking in rational nature' (*naturae rationalis individua substantia*), was quoted by the moralists throughout the centuries.[10] In the period of cellular cleavage, before the embryo is formed, individuality is not yet. A person has yet to be.

The aim of this chapter has been, not to claim contemporary relevance for either an outmoded embryology or an outmoded philosophical speculation on the soul and the time of its 'entering' (if it does) the body; nor yet to ventilate again the liceity of abortion. It has been to recall a moral tradition *expressed in terms* of these three things, persisting to the end of the nineteenth century, and, for those cognisant of the arcane casuistry of medical practice, beyond that date unto this day. The tradition attempted to grade the protection accorded to the nascent human being according to the stages of its development. The tradition is challenged today by those who claim absolute protection 'from the moment of conception' and so would forbid forms of post-coital contraception (like the hormonal compounds or intra-uterine devices) which inhibit implantation, and any use of ova fertilised *in vitro* not directed towards their being implanted and brought to term in live birth.

The motive prompting the restriction is admirable: to resist the erosion of the value of human life, already savagely assailed in the world's present economic and political activities. But we have to choose. Uterine life must be protected at some point. If we put that point too early, forbidding observation and experimental use of pre-implantation embryos in the early stages of cell division, we shall inhibit much useful research of potential human benefit including the improvement of the chances of successful pregnancy for lack of which many extra embryos are sacrificed at present. Embryologists themselves search for means of determining a point beyond which experiment would be intolerable; some would relate that point to the emergence of the primitive streak on the embryonic plate, when individuality begins; others to the beginning of the development of the nervous system, anticipating the capacity of the fetus for sensitivity or awareness – words used by Dante, as we have seen, as characteristic of the fetus so grown as to warrant the attribution of rational, human soul. Knowledge in embryology may change; but perhaps there are aspects of human relating to it which are perennial.

References and notes

1 Catholic Social Welfare Commission. *Human fertilization: choices for the future.* Evidence of the Catholic Social Welfare Commission to the Government Enquiry into Human Fertilization and Embryology. Abingdon, CSWC, 1983: s 43, p 21.
2 J Mahoney. *Bioethics and belief.* London, Sheed and Ward, 1984.
3 N M Ford. *When did I begin?* Cambridge, Cambridge University Press, 1988.
4 A Chollet. Animation. In: A Vacant and E Mangenot (eds) *Dictionnaire de théologie Catholique.* Paris, Latouzey et Ane, 1903: col 1305 ff.
5 J Delmaille. Avortement. In: R Naz (ed) *Dictionnaire de droit canonique.* Paris, Latouzey et Ane, 1938: col 1536 ff.
6 G R Driver and J C Miles. *The Babylonian laws,* Oxford, Clarendon Press, 1953: II, pp 209–214.

7 S M Paul. *The book of the Covenant*, 1965. Quoted by: J R Hyatt. *Commentary on Exodus*, 1971: p 233.

8 H E Sigerist. *A history of medicine*. Oxford, Oxford University Press, 1951: I, p 430.

9 I Jacobovits. *Jewish medical ethics*. New York, Bloch, 1975: p 372.

10 Thomas de Chobham (1216). *See* F Broomfield (ed) *Thomae de Chobham Summa Confessorum*. Louvain, Editions Nauwellaerts, 1968: pp 49, 463 f.

11 Hippocrates. *See* Nutriment, XLII. In: W H S Jones (ed) *The Hippocratic writings*. Loeb Classics, 1923: I.

12 Aristotle. *See* J A Smith (translator) *De anima*. In: W D Ross (ed) *The works of Aristotle*. Oxford, Clarendon Press, 1931: III, pp 402a6 ff.

13 Aristotle. *See* D M Balme (ed) *De generatione animalium*. Oxford, Clarendon Press, 1972: pp 731a25, 734b4 ff.

14 Aristotle. *See* D Wentworth Thompson (ed) *Historia animalium*. In: J F Smith and D Ross (eds) *The works of Aristotle*. Oxford, Clarendon Press, 1910: IV, pp VII, 3, 583b. (For help in relating this reference to St Thomas on *The Sentences* I am indebted to Dr Roland Hall of the University of York.)

15 L Bieler. *The Irish penitentials*. Dublin, Institute for Advanced Studies, 1963: pp 160, 228, 474.

16 F Schulz. Bracton and Raymond de Penafort. *Law Quarterly Review*, 1xi, 1945: p 288.

17 L C Hector and B F Harvey (eds) *The Westminster chronicle, 1381–1394*. Oxford, Oxford University Press, 1982: pp 322 f.

18 G L Bickersteth. *Dante Alighieri: the divine comedy*. Oxford, Basil Blackwell, 1972. (See also translator's note on p 790.)

19 C Grobstein. External human fertilization. *Scientific American*, 240, 1979: pp 33–43.

20 C Grobstein. *From change to purpose: an appraisal of external human fertilization*. London, Addison Wesley, 1981.

21 C Horstmann (ed) *The early south east legendary or lives of the saints*. London, Early English Text Society, 1887: Original series 87, p 319 ff.

22 T Vicary. *The anatomie of the bodie of man*. First published 1548, republished and revised by his colleagues at St Bartholomew's Hospital in 1577. F J Furnivall and P Furnivall (eds) London, Oxford University Press for the Early English Text Society, ES LIII 1888, second impression 1930.

57

6

EXPERIMENT ON HUMAN EMBRYOS: SENTIENCE AS THE CUT-OFF POINT?

John Marshall

Some of those who advocate experimenting on human embryos propose as a cut-off point emergence of the ability to feel pain. The proposition is usually put in the form: of course experiment should not continue beyond the point at which the embryo can feel pain. The purpose of this paper is to examine some of the philosophical and biological implications of this stance.

Pain is a subjective experience. No one can feel another person's pain. Our sympathy with a person in pain derives entirely by analogy from our own experience. Much effort has been devoted to making the measurement of pain more objective but with little success. The pain producing stimulus can be carefully quantified but the recipient's experience of it cannot.

The subjective experience of pain has objective corre-lates. The tightened lips, the wince, the cry or scream are examples of this. Physiological phenomena such as pulse rate, blood pressure, and constriction of blood vessels are also affected and can be measured. But these measures are not of the severity of the pain but of the person's reaction to it. The pharmacological substances known as endorphins in the brain play an important role in this and are the subject of increasing study and experiment. But in the final analysis, pain remains a subjective experience.

Though pain itself cannot be measured, we can at least note the objective correlates and use them as a kind of albeit imperfect measure. This is not entirely satisfactory. We may assume that when a certain stimulus, which our experience tells us is painful, is applied to another human being or to another species, the recipient feels pain. We may also assume that the severity of the pain is reflected in the degree of the response. These assumptions are not always justified. If, for example, a painful stimulus is applied to the foot of a paraplegic person, there will be vigorous withdrawal of the limb as though it had been hurt but the person feels no pain; the withdrawal is entirely reflex. Observing a response to a painful stimulus does not justify the conclusion that the recipient even feels pain, let alone provide a measure of its severity.

Turning now to the situation relating to the embryo we must first look at the development of the nervous structures which subserve the experience of pain. The neural tube folds at about 21 days after fertilisation, and the first sign of a cerebral cortex appears at about six weeks, with a major proliferation of brain cells at eight weeks. The appearance of a structure does not, however, indicate that it is immediately functional. For example, though brain cells appear at eight weeks, connections between them are not established until much later. However, movement patterns which imply considerable interconnections within the nervous system can be seen by 14 weeks.

There is no means of knowing at what point in the development of its nervous system the embryo can feel pain. To circumvent this difficulty the appearance of the necessary nervous structures could be taken as a prudent cut-off point even though they may not yet be functional. Is this a sufficient safeguard? Organisms without a neural structure respond to stimulation. Even simple cellular organisms react quite vigorously to noxious stimuli. Can it be said that they feel pain? Can we rest secure in the view that we need not be concerned about the ability of the human embryo to feel pain prior to the emergence of the nervous system?

In summary, taking the ability to feel pain as the cut-off point for experiment on human embryos abounds with difficulty at the biological level. The appearance of neural structures does not indicate that the embryo can feel pain; the structures may as yet be functionless. On the other hand, the absence of neural structures does not mean that

59

the embryo must be unresponsive to painful stimuli. Neural development is therefore a signpost which may give comfort to the experimenter but provides little in the way of hard evidence as to the experience of the embryo. It would therefore be a very unsatisfactory criterion by which to determine a cut-off point for experiment on the human embryo.

Turning to the philosophical aspects, why is sentience so important that it is proferred as a cut-off point? The simple answer is of an axiomatic nature: to inflict pain is wrong. This applies even to animals. Man slaughters animals for food, but civilised societies go to great lengths to ensure that the slaughter is painless and humane. Experiment on animals is strictly controlled by law and painful procedures must be carried out under anaesthesia. No matter how great the knowledge to be gained by an animal experiment this does not justify the infliction of unnecessary pain.

The same argument can be applied to experiment on embryos. No experiment should be carried out which would involve inflicting pain. This may be axiomatic but immed-iately raises another question. If it is simply that pain must not be inflicted, then a technical advance which enabled the embryo or fetus to be anaesthetised, as are human beings after birth, would remove the cut-off point. Experiments could then presumably continue to a new cut-off point determined by some other criterion.

The ability of the human embryo to feel pain cannot be taken as a satisfactory cut-off point for experiment. Apart from the prognostic difficulty in establishing where to place that point, the use of this criterion is in effect an evasion of the real issue. Experiments on and slaughter of animals are permitted provided that pain is not caused. To allow experiments on human embryos before they are considered capable of feeling pain would be to adopt the same criterion as we do for animals. Is this in fact what we are doing by proposing that experiments on the human embryo should be allowed up to the point at which it might feel pain? Are we denying it any status that is peculiarly human?

The use of this criterion is in effect a form of escapism.

By saying that pain must not be inflicted, which appears as a praiseworthy moral stance, the fact escapes notice that no answer is being given to the important question of the status of the human embryo. If the embryo is thought to be a person, in the sense of someone who cannot be used as a means to an end, the fact that what is being done can be done without pain becomes an irrelevance. The question, what is being done, must be faced. Is what is being done compatible with the status of the embryo as a person or potential person? This is the question to be answered, not whether or not the embryo will feel pain. The latter question is an evasion of the former question to which this book is addressed.

7

THE STATUS OF THE EMBRYO IN THE JEWISH TRADITION

Sir Immanuel Jakobovits

The criteria determining the status of the embryo in Jewish law and thought are varied, and the relevant opinions of authentic teachers are by no means monolithic. But on one fundamental principle there is complete agreement: full human status is not acquired until birth, and until then the destruction of a product of conception does not constitute homicide culpable as murder.

In fact, the determination of the embryo's status, or perhaps rather non-status, derives primarily from the laws of murder, at least in their biblical formulation. Bloodshed is a captial offence for the express reason that man was made in the Divine Image (*Genesis* 9:6). However, in the law revealed at Sinai, such guilt is limited to the killing of 'a man' (*Exodus* 21:12; *Leviticus* 24:17). Jewish exegesis interprets this as 'a man – but not an unborn child'. Accordingly, the destruction of a fetus, resulting from an attack on a pregnant mother, carries a monetary liability for the payment of damages (*Exodus* 21:22), and such monetary obligation is always excluded in cases of capital acts. All these passages clearly exempt feticide from the laws of murder, and they therefore firmly refuse to establish full human status before birth.

Parenthetically, it might be mentioned here that the parting of the ways between the Jewish and the Christian traditions has its origin in the differing versions or translations of the *Exodus* passage on assaulting a pregnant mother. While the Hebrew text, as authentically interpreted in the earliest rabbinic commentaries, applies the crucial words 'if there be no accident' to the mother surviving the assault, the Septuagint (evidently based on a variant Samaritan reading or simply on a mistranslation) renders these words 'if it be without form', that is, if the fetus has not yet assumed human shape, thus exempting the attacker from capital liability only up to that stage of fetal development, but making him liable to the death penalty for the destruction of the fetus thereafter. This position was maintained by the early Church Fathers and later upheld for many centuries until the distinction between formed and unformed fetuses was eventually eliminated to treat as murder the destruction of any germinating human life from the moment of conception, an attitude maintained by the Catholic Church in principle to the present day.

Returning to Jewish sources, once the embryo is denied full human status, the definition of its remaining 'rights' is complex, and authentic rabbinic opinions are often considerably at variance with each other.

Again, agreement unites virtually all authorities only in conferring some degree of protection on the embryo from the moment of conception until birth in various stages of increasing human identity. In part, this identity is without any intrinsic autonomy. For instance, some schools in the Talmud speak of the fetus in certain legal contexts merely as 'a limb of the mother', not treated as a separate entity, corresponding to *pars viscerum matris* in Roman law. Indeed, several later authorities object to a non-therapeutic abortion only as an extension of the prohibition against 'spilling the seed in vain'. This severe interdict (of what is loosely called Onanism) is itself merely the obverse of the biblical precept to 'be fruitful and multiply' (*Genesis* 1:28; 9:1), that is, as implying a prohibition on frustrating the procreative act.

Again, some authorities in the Talmud deem the embryo during the first forty days following conception 'as mere water', but the context in which this particular formulation occurs deals only with the levitical laws of impurity normally following a birth or a miscarriage (*Leviticus* 12:1–5). Nevertheless, as we shall see, some later decisors use this source for adopting the most lenient attitude to abortions carried out during the first forty days – in other words, for attributing the least 'rights' or status to this initial period in the life of an embryo.

Two indirect references, though of no legal consequence whatever, may appear to have some bearing on the place of the embryo in Jewish thought. The Talmud ascribes certain spiritual attributes to children before birth. For instance, babes in their mothers' womb are said to have joined in the Song of Moses and the Children of Israel after their safe deliverance from the Egyptians at the Red Sea. Similarly, they were a party to the Covenant sworn between God and Israel at Sinai and on entering the Land of Israel. Into the same category of practically inconsequential, yet theologically not insignificant statements, belongs the argument reported in the Talmud between the Roman Emperor Antoninus and Rabbi Judah, the compiler of the Mishnah, on the entry of the soul, with the Rabbi eventually conceding that this must occur at the time of conception rather than (as he had originally held) on the embryo's assumption of human form or on its physical completion at birth, and this revised opinion was supported by the verse 'and Your visitation has preserved my spirit' (*Job* 10:12). Interesting as these passages may be in theory, they have never been used in practice to determine the status of the embryo in Jewish law.

Far more relevant, and yet not entirely conclusive, as an indicator of embryonic 'rights' or status is the rule on the suspension of the Sabbath laws if their observance would cause the slightest risk to life. Whether this suspension rule also applies to the saving of a fetal life *in utero* if otherwise deemed to be at risk is not expressly treated in the Talmud itself, except in the case of a mother who died in childbirth when permission was given for the Sabbath to be violated in an effort to rescue her child by a Caesarian operation. However, it is only among medieval and later rabbis that consideration was given to the violation of the Sabbath rules expressly for the sake of a fetus otherwise in danger during an earlier stage of gestation. Some permitted this specifically out of regard for the life of the unborn child, but others contemplated setting aside the Sabbath law for a fetus only because any risk to its life might also endanger the mother for whose safety the Sabbath would certainly have to give way.

But there are reservations in conclusions on the status of the embryo to be drawn from the readiness of the rabbis to rule leniently on the Sabbath laws when these might conflict with the safety of fetal life, inasmuch as the normal Sabbath regulations demand their suspension in the face of not only a definite and grave threat to life but of even a remote risk.

As against these last-mentioned sources, which clearly attach some significant status to the fetus demanding protection, there are others which tend in the opposite direction. For instance, in discussing the fate of a pregnant woman sentenced to death (however hypothetical this is, in view of the virtual abolition of capital punishment in Jewish law some two thousand years ago), the Talmud weighs two conflicting interests: the child's in being delivered before the execution, and the mother's in not having the agony of suspense between the sentence and its execution drawn out. The decision is in favour of the mother at the expense of the unborn child, unless the process of birth had already begun. In that case, the child is regarded as 'a separate body', and the sentence is not carried out until after the birth is complete. By the same token of disregarding the fetus as an entity separate from the mother until birth, the conversion to Judaism of a pregnant mother (completed by her immersion in a ritual bath) automatically includes the child on being born, and its Jewish status is established without any further ceremony. Based on the same reasoning of legal non-status, a fetus cannot acquire things, and the assignment of any gift or property to an unborn child is invalid, except when made by its own father (because – to interpret the relevant source rather broadly – in the father's subjective mind his child constitutes a real person with consequent legal rights even before birth).

None of these opinions or rulings provides absolutely

65

conclusive evidence for the status of prenatal life in Jewish law; indeed, some are quite marginal or altogether irrelevant. Moreover, these judgments, while they usually represent a consensus of rabbinic opinion, are by no means universally endorsed. In most cases, they are subject to considerable arguments, and often to reservations and variations in matters of detail which could not be listed here. What does emerge quite distinctly is, on the one hand, a refusal to grant full human inviolability to the unborn child from conception and, on the other hand, clear recognition that the potentiality for life must not be compromised except for the most substantial medical reasons.

It is only in the more recent writings of the rabbinical responsa (that is, written and usually published collections of verdicts on Jewish law by leading rabbinical scholars) that we find the status of the embryo defined in terms directly applicable to the current debate. These are notably in the form of answers to enquiries on abortions at different stages of gestation and in varying circumstances in the grey area between a life-hazard to the mother and some lesser concern for the welfare of the mother or the normality of the child to be born. These practical conclusions are quite often unrelated to the assertion or negation of fetal entitlements mentioned earlier.

What we have, then, are several somewhat vaguely distinct stages in the evolving status of the embryo. During the first forty days following conception the embryo is generally regarded as 'mere water' and lacking any specifically human 'rights', at least in the view of most authorities. At this stage its inviolability derives purely from its potential growth into a human being, not from its actual endowment of human qualities, however rudimentary or as yet infinitesimal. The destruction of such a germinating conceptus is therefore not essentially different from the deliberate wastage of male semen. Both are condemned as grave offences, and perhaps even as appurtenances of murder, but only in a figurative sense. But there is certainly no distinction made between the first two weeks and the remainder of the forty-day period.

66

The next stage, according to the consensus of rabbinic opinion, takes the embryo up to the end of the third month, when human form is established and becomes visible on the expulsion or extraction of the embryo. During this stage the embryo's life is more strictly protected in the sense that the indications for its destruction would have to be graver than in the earlier stage; for instance, the risk to the mother or of the child being born with abnormalities would need to be rated correspondingly higher for the pregnancy to be interrupted.

However, some authorities extend this stage even up to and including the seventh month, provided the considerations for an abortion are urgent enough. For example, if an amniocentesis cannot be carried out during the earlier stage, and there are reasons to suspect genetic or congenital abnormalities in the child, these authorities would favour a lenient view right into the seventh month, even though viability of a premature birth could be established before then.

The final prenatal stage, when the fetus assumes a quasi-human status, is during parturition, that is, when the birth process has actually started and the fetus has 'dislodged itself from its uterine moorings'. It is then regarded not yet as a separate life, but as 'a separate body', to the extent that its destruction at this stage could be sanctioned only by applying the 'aggressor' argument, that is, if the fetus posed a direct threat to the life of the mother, for instance, by a breach birth which cannot be delivered without a grave hazard to the mother. Following in particular the Code of Maimonides, the inferior status of the unborn child would then no longer be sufficient by itself to warrant its destruction for the sake of the mother without recourse to the special law of 'pursuit' which demands the elimination of anyone threatening an innocent human life.

Biblical sources and major principles

To facilitate the reader in linking the principal relevant considerations in Jewish law with their biblical origins, it may be helpful at this point to list these sources and then to define the considerations derived from them:

Man's creation 'in the image of God' (*Genesis* 1:27) confers infinite value on every innocent human life and renders its destruction into a capital offence. While this absolute inviolability – whereby no life may ever be deliberately sacrified even to save another or any number of others – sets in only at birth (*Exodus* 21:12, 22–23, and Jewish commentaries). The unborn child, too, enjoys a very sacred title to life, in different stages from the moment of conception, to be set aside only in exceptional circumstances, such as a serious hazard to the mother.

Judaism lists the duty of procreation ('Be fruitful and multiply' – *Genesis* 1:28; 9:1) as the first of its 613 Commandments. Conversely, it deems the destruction of the human seed as a grave violation of this law. While Judaism therefore sets the highest value and importance on the fulfilment of marriage through children (see *Genesis* 30:31), it sanctions the generation of life exclusively through the bonds sanctified by marriage.

Judaism's strict code of sexual morality, especially the laws on incest (*Leviticus* 18:1–30; 20:8–27), presupposes that the (biological) father and mother of a child are known and can be identified with absolute certainty. No legal contract or artificial act can suspend, override or replace natural relationships based on consanguinity.

The duty to preserve human life and health is a religious precept (*Deuteronomy* 4:9, 15), which includes the Divine sanction to intervene in the course of nature or Providence by the practice of medicine (*Exodus* 21:19). But this sanction conferred on doctors is limited to acts of healing, or procedures intended to serve therapeutic ends.

Man, created to 'hold dominion over the fish of the sea and the birds of the heavens and every living thing crawling on the earth' (*Genesis* 1:28), is entitled to exploit animals in his service and for his health, provided they are protected from all avoidable suffering.

From these basic postulates derive the following general guidelines germane to the issues related to the status of the embryo, notably in the treatment of infertility and experiments on embryos:

Society is under an obligation to promote the moral and physical health of its members. To this end, medical science should harness human ingenuity and all available resources in the battle against disease and physical disabilities, including infertility, so long as this is done without infringing overriding moral imperatives, such as to uphold the sanctity of life, the dignity of every individual, the inviolability of marriage and the distinctiveness of all natural species.

The erosion of the family founded on marriage, as the basic unit of society, is a greater social and moral evil threatening the stability of society and its fundamental values than the suffering of individuals caused by disease or childlessness. Hence, relief from such suffering must never be purchased at the cost of impairing the sanctity of marriage and its function as the sole legitimate agency for the procreation of children.

More important than to produce children is to secure conditions under which they will be raised by parents in homes providing love and compassionate care. To deprive children of this security even before they are born is a betrayal of our human trust and responsibility. Moreover, it is every child's inalienable birthright to have identifiable natural parents, even if sometimes their identity is not publicly divulged or given to the child himself, as in cases of adoption. In these exceptional circumstances, the parentage must still be carefully recorded, with such privileged information being made available to specialised agencies for the prevention of incestuous unions or on other legitimate grounds in the interests of the child.

When the sperm and the ovum are taken exclusively from a husband and his wife, there is no essential difference in principle between *in vitro* fertilisation (IVF) and artificial insemination from the husband (AIH), but the controls to guard against the possible admixture or confusion of the vital cells from other donors, whether deliberately or by mistake, require special surveillance, possibly by two independent supervisors. The sanction of IVF must pass every reasonable test to avoid any undue risk to the mother and possible damage to the embryo before applying the procedure to an otherwise infertile marriage.

The destruction of an unborn child, let alone of an embryo in the earlier stages of gestation, does not constitute murder, since the unqualified entitlement to life – equal to the claim to inviolability of any other human being – sets in only at birth. Nevertheless, the germinating product of conception enjoys a very sacred title to life which may be set aside by deliberate destruction or abortion only in the most exceptional cases of medical urgency, notably to save the life of the mother if this would otherwise be at risk.

There is no moral objection in principle to genetic engineering or manipulation, provided such deliberate interference with the building-blocks of life serves exclusively well-tested therapeutic purposes to eliminate physical or mental defects caused by hereditary or genetic disorders. On animals, the sanction for such manipulation also includes experiments or procedures designed to advance human health and nutrition.

In all these operations on human genes, the critical difference is between 'improving' nature and correcting it (or between positive and negative eugenics). The elimination of any abnormality or defect to ensure the health of children to be born is morally no different from any other medical or surgical intervention to overcome nature's disabilities. Such acts of healing, whether performed on organs, limbs or genes, are included in the biblical sanction or dispensation granted to doctors. But this licence does not cover acts of intervention in nature lacking therapeutic justification. The ecological arguments against undue interference with man's environment are infinitely increased against such interference with man himself. So are the dangers that may result from such intervention by possibly adding to each successive generation the cumulative effect of impairing nature's checks and balances.

Thus the cloning of human beings or the predetermination of their sex before birth might well lead eventually to a preponderance of, for instance, intellectuals or males, which could destroy the delicately-balanced fabric of society. Man has neither the right nor the competence to compete with nature, or Providence, in its preserves.

The only circumstances under which the freezing of gametes could be morally justified are the imminent likelihood of a parent becoming unable to consummate a conception, such as a husband about to undergo radiological treatment or a wife anticipating an operation on her ovaries. But freezing procedures for longer periods, especially for posthumous use, should be strongly opposed, and the notion of a 'storage authority' is altogether repugnant.

Experimenting on human embryos

Some of the arguments advanced against experimenting on human embryos seem quite irrelevant or unconvincing. For instance, the embryo's inability to give informed consent is as immaterial an impediment as 'the balance of . . . pleasure over pain' or being 'incapable of feeling pain' can determine the ethics of experiments on embryos. Human rights or their absence cannot be related to any of these criteria which are completely extrinsic to inviolability. What is crucial in allowing the use of embryos for experiments is that they must have been brought into being not for research purposes but solely for the possible prospect of ensuring a successful pregnancy. The moment they are no longer potentially required, or in a fit condition, for possible reimplantation, no further experiments should be done; until then, such observation or tests as do not necessarily lead to their destruction (by irreversible damage to them) may be carried out. What matters, therefore, is not any arbitrary time span, but the motive for their generation and their potential for reimplantation.

71

The difficulty of defining the circumstances, if any, in which experiments and research may be carried out on *in vitro* embryos is fully recognised. None but 'spares' could be so used in exceptional cases, and then only if certain conditions (such as are set out in the Warnock report) are met. But the arbitrary fourteen-day limit should be replaced by the proviso that such 'spares' should only be used or preserved if and when it is feasible to reimplant them in the mother with the prospect of normal development to a live birth.

The family and the child

The two other considerations overriding the more limited question of the embryo's rights and status concern the stability of the family and the essential interests of the child to be born. Both these considerations may be of more far-reaching consequence for promoting the essential foundations of the moral order than defining the precise point at which human life with its absolute value commences. This priority in the Jewish scale of concerns will be reflected in the presentation of attitudes and judgments on the wide diversity of issues raised by the progress of medical science and techniques.

A direct result of man's capacity to supplant the natural generation of life is the threat to the family. The concern for its stability, let alone its inviolability as the exclusive agency for the creation of children, seems to be almost abandoned by some proposals on artificial insemination and fertilisation. It appears no longer a matter of urgent public policy to safeguard the most essential unit of the social fabric. By expressly dissociating the definition of a 'couple' from a legal husband–wife relationship and by legalising the false entry of AID and IVF children as born to parents who are in fact infertile, these proposals would turn marriage into an acceptable casualty of technological progress. Such indifference to mankind's oldest and most vital institution can only compound the havoc already created by the debris of broken homes on a colossal scale.

72

Another cardinal imperative in regulating the generation of human life is the overriding insistence on the interests of the child. It is an indefensible violation of rights which should be deemed inalienable to engage in such practices as, for example, the deliberate creation of orphans (by freezing semen, eggs or embryos for possible use after the donor's death); the permanent deception of children on their paternity (by AID and the fraudulent entry of the mother's barren husband as the father); or conceiving children by one mother to be borne by another (as a 'surrogate'), with the prospect that both may one day lay conflicting claims to the child. (Indeed, some rabbinic authorities would deem the host-mother to be the child's legal parent if transplantation occurred before the fetus was viable, since they regard maternal identity to be established at parturition rather than at conception.[1]) Altogether, to raise children who will never be able to identify for certain their immediate ancestry nor their closest blood-relations is an affront to human dignity as well as to the moral order. Children facing the trauma of such shocking conflicts and uncertainties on seeking their origins are at a grave disadvantage in building socially and morally stable lives.

Reference

1 J David Bleich. Medical genetics: commentary. *New York State Journal of Medicine*, August 1982: p 1374.

8

ROMAN CATHOLIC CASUISTRY AND THE MORAL STANDING OF THE HUMAN EMBRYO

Brendan Soane

Introduction

Casuistry is the application of general moral principles to particular cases. How do Roman Catholics apply the moral principles governing the sanctity of human life to the treatment of human embryos? In fact, as I hope to show, not all Roman Catholics are in agreement. Those who speak officially on behalf of the Roman Catholic communion propose one teaching but a number of Catholic scholars, speaking in their own name, disagree with it to a greater or lesser degree. I will outline the official teaching before dealing with divergent views.

Before doing so it will be useful to say a few words about the current state of Catholic moral theology. There are three major controversies among Catholic scholars which bear on our topic. The first concerns the relationship between official teaching, which is enunciated by those who are entrusted with the pastoral care of the Church, that is, the Pope and the other bishops, and the teaching of theologians. To what extent ought a theologian to feel free, while still acting as a Catholic theologian, to dissent from official teaching, and what standing has his teaching if he does? Can it be considered Catholic teaching, or is it merely a private opinion? The issue is particularly acute when it is a question of scholars who work in Catholic universities and seminaries. Understandably, many theologians put a less restrictive interpretation on their professional role than do some who hold office in the Church. This controversy is important because it specifies what is meant by Roman Catholic in my title. The meaning which one gives it will depend on one's understanding of teaching authority in the Church.

The second controversy concerns the sources of Christian moral teaching. Are there specifically Christian ethics? If there are not, and some Catholic scholars claim that this is the case, then moral norms must be based on rational considerations alone, the sort of considerations discussed by Byrne in this volume. But if there are specifically Christian ethics, then we must seek in divine revelation for at least some of the considerations which will help us to form our moral judgments. Rational considerations alone will not suffice. It is not necessarily the case that those who believe that there are specifically Christian ethics will favour official teaching and those who believe ethics to be autonomous will favour change. Some scholars argue in favour of official positions on purely rational grounds. But belief about this issue will determine how one goes about the task of seeking moral norms. It will also affect any readiness to dialogue with non-Christians with the expectation of reaching a consensus. If ethics are thought of as autonomous there will be more hope of reaching agreement in a group like that which produced this volume.

The third controversy concerns the absoluteness of moral norms. In recent years a number of scholars have questioned the received teaching that the moral prohibition of certain actions, such as the direct killing of innocent human beings, direct sterilisation, contraception and abortion, is without exception. The debate focuses on the extent to which foreseen consequences have a bearing on the judgment as to whether a proposed act is morally licit. That too will affect judgment about the treatment of embryos. Is the moral norm prohibiting taking innocent human life an absolute covering all human life from fertilisation to death, or is the embryo a special case which could justify destructive experiments for a sufficiently good reason?

These controversies are as yet unresolved. Since this is so one cannot enunciate a body of Catholic teaching about the human embryo in the secure confidence that it is complete and fixed. It is still developing, in response to new questions, new scientific data and new insights, both about the embryo and about Christian ethics. But development will never be so great that new teaching will be sharply discontinuous with the past. Christianity is not just a body of truths, but a way of life, and that way of life is not going to change radically. Attitudes to human life, to marriage and the family, to the Creator and His creation, will develop, but they will not change so much as to be discontinuous. I do not think, for example, that the main lines of Catholic teaching on abortion will change. It might happen that the embryo will be seen to be a special case, and that non-therapeutic experiments on embryos will be found to be acceptable, Personally, I do not think a sufficiently strong case has been made out to justify such a change in teaching. I think respect for human life demands that we refrain from harm and do only good from fertilisation on, whatever benefits experiment may seem to offer mankind. I think this is so even though the status of the early embryo is uncertain. It may not be an individual, but it shares our common humanity and is on the way to becoming an individual if permitted to do so.

Historical background

John R Connery SJ, in a historical study of the Catholic teaching on abortion, shows that Catholic teaching has always condemned abortion from the time of conception onwards.[1] It was not always taught that the fetus was a human person from the time of conception. A distinction was made between fetuses which had not yet received a human form and those which had (unformed and formed fetuses). Another distinction was made between those which did not yet have a human soul and those which had (unensouled or unanimated and ensouled or animated). These distinctions did not necessarily coincide. It was possible to hold at one and the same time that the soul was given at the time of conception and that the fetus was not formed until much later. But most authors seem to have held that ensoulment and formation (about forty days for boys and eighty for girls) coincided.

76

These distinctions did not have a major importance for moral judgment. It must be remembered that sterilisation (by castration) and contraception were considered grave sins, and for much of the history of the Church it was taught that they shared the malice of homicide. The canon law recognised the distinction between killing a fetus before and after ensoulment by imposing a larger penance in the latter case. But there were penances attached to sterilisation, contraception and abortion at any stage of fetal development.

Casuistry made its mark in the late middle ages. A number of theologians defended the opinion that, whereas in the normal course of events it would be immoral to expel a fetus at any stage of its development, if the fetus were a threat to the mother's life it was morally lawful to abort it, but only if it were not yet ensouled. This opinion was defended by many theologians, though never by all, from the fourteenth to the seventeenth centuries, when it fell into abeyance. Meanwhile, following a suggestion by a theologian called Antonius de Corduba (1485–1578) it became a common opinion that one might apply life-saving remedies to a mother who was in danger of death even though they were indirectly a danger to the life of the fetus. This is accepted and taught in the Catholic Church today. Catholic teaching permits indirect abortion for a proportionate reason but not direct abortion. There is direct abortion when abortion is sought as an end in itself or a means to another end. There is indirect abortion when it results from some other therapeutic procedure.

Recent authoritative teaching

Popes and bishops today teach that the life of the human person must be inviolate from the time of conception. For example, Pope Paul VI in an allocution to Italian Jurists in 1973 said that the state's protection of human life should begin at conception, '... this being the beginning of a new human being'.[2]

Richard McCormick SJ, writing in *Theological Studies* in

1974[3], said that there was total unanimity in the recent teaching of the Pope and bishops that the right to life began at conception. Human life is seen as a continuum. Typical of this way of thinking was the statement of the Catholic Archbishops of Great Britain in 1980.[4] They alluded to the phenomenon of twinning but went on to say ' . . . from the time of conception, the features which distinguish us from each of our parents . . . are laid down in the "genetic code" that comes into existence then. Each such new life is the life not of a potential human being but of a human being with potential. The development of this potential is normally a process of profound continuity.'[5]

These teachings do not pretend to settle the age-old dispute about the time of ensoulment. They are of a practical nature, saying what may and may not be done to a human fetus. When the Sacred Congregation for the Doctrine of the Faith issued a statement on procured abortion in 1974, they explicitly declared that they were not touching on the question of the moment of ensoulment and that the moral issue of the condemnation of abortion from the time of conception did not depend on the solution to this problem. They argued that even if the soul should be infused some time after conception 'nonetheless in the fetus was a human life beginning . . . which prepares for and demands a human soul through which the nature received from the parents is perfected . . . even if the infusion of that soul should be judged only probable (for the matter can never be established) to repress the life is the same as to take the risk of killing a man, not merely in spe, but already informed by a soul.'[6]

The Sacred Congregation considered the presence or absence of a soul a question for philosophy which could not be settled by scientific study. Hence the parenthesis (non enim de re unquam constabit), 'for the matter can never be established'. But the question of what to do is a moral question, and that should be settled in favour of the life of the fetus, otherwise one would risk killing a human being.

It is not usually the task of the teaching authority to settle cases of conscience. But on the matter of abortion we find examples of the application of general principles to particular cases. For example, the statement of the Archbishops of England and Wales which was quoted above devotes a paragraph to the case of rape. It includes the following passage:

A woman is certainly entitled to defend herself against the continuing effects of such an attack and to seek immediate medical assistance with a view to preventing conception. In a very small number of cases, conception may in fact occur. Then there exists a new being whose individuality, distinct from each of its parents and from any of their cells, we have already described. From that time, the requirements of the moral law, transcending even the most understandable emotional reactions, are clear; the newly-conceived child cannot rightly be made to suffer the penalty of death for a man's violation of the woman.[7]

More recently Pope John Paul II addressed himself to experiments on human embryos. To a gathering of biologists in Vatican City on 23 October 1982, he said:

I have no reason to be apprehensive for those experiments in biology which are performed by scientists, who, like you, have a profound respect for the human person, since I am sure that they will contribute to the integral well-being of man. On the other hand, I condemn, in the most explicit and formal way, experimental manipulations of the human embryo, since the human being, from conception to death, cannot be exploited for any purpose whatsoever.[8]

A recent instruction from the Sacred Congregation for the Doctrine of the Faith has reaffirmed the same teaching.[9] While acknowledging that the Church teaching office has not committed itself to an affirmation of a philosophical nature concerning the presence or otherwise of a spiritual soul in the human embryo, it reaffirms the moral condemnation of any kind of procured abortion. It claims that this teaching is unchangeable. It goes on to say that from the

79

moment the zygote is formed it demands the unconditional respect that is morally due to the human being in his bodily and spiritual totality, it must be respected and treated as a person and its rights must be recognised. The instruction goes on to condemn among other practices non-therapeutic experiments on human embryos, the production of embryos destined to be exploited as disposable 'biological material', the voluntary destruction of human embryos obtained for the sole purpose of research, exposing such embryos to death, the freezing of embryos and attempts to influence chromosomic or genetic inheritance.

Theological opinion

The task of theologians is to explore and to question within the Christian tradition. They do not simply repeat what bishops say but attempt to develop Church teaching by bringing it to bear on cases and by confronting it with new knowledge from whatever source. Some theologians are content in the matter of the treatment of human embryos simply to repeat without question the teaching of Church authorities, and to draw logical conclusions. An example of this was the evidence submitted to the Warnock committee by the Catholic Bishops' Joint Committee on Bio-Ethical Issues. (The Committee was set up by the bishops of England, Wales and Scotland, and has been extended to represent the Irish hierarchy. It includes a number of bishops and other specialists.) This committee was of the belief that a number of practices connected with *in vitro* fertilisation are 'fundamentally unacceptable and ought to be prohibited in any civilised community'. These included:

> 11.1 Any form of experimentation on a human embryo which is likely to damage that embryo, or to endanger it by delaying the time of its transfer and implantation, other than procedures intended to benefit the embryo itself;
> 11.2 Any form of observation of a human embryo which damages that human embryo, or endangers it by delaying the time of its transfer and implantation, other than

observations made for the benefit of that embryo itself;
11.3 Any form of freezing or other storage without genuine or definite prospect of subsequent transfer, unimpaired, to the proper mother;
11.4 Any form of selection among living and developing human embryos, with a view to transferring and implanting only the fittest or most desirable.[10]

A majority of this committee would also have wished to judge *in vitro* fertilisation itself morally illicit, although that was not a unanimous opinion.

Teaching very similar to that of this committee has since been promulgated by the Congregation for the Doctrine of the Faith in its Instruction of 22 February 1987, including the condemnation of *in vitro* fertilisation; this latter on the grounds that it is contrary to the dignity of procreation and the conjugal union.

The remainder of the paper will be concerned with more exploratory views which have no official standing, but are the views of reputable theologians. Rather than refer to individual writers I will simply summarise the sorts of view which are found in the literature.

The most important question at issue is that of when the developing embryo becomes a human person. In seeking to answer that question Catholic writers usually appeal to criteria intrinsic to the developing embryo, rather than to extrinsic criteria, such as, for example, the acceptance of the developing person by other persons.

One way of asking the question is the traditional one of asking when the soul is infused. At what stage of biological development does the embryo receive a soul? Some say at the time of fertilisation. Others suggest that individuation must be complete and twinning no longer possible. Others argue for more development than that. They may require that the nervous system be present in outline, or that the basic structure of the cerebral cortex be established. Others avoid the language of souls and ensoulment, but give a similar range of answers to the question of when the embryo becomes a person.

Whatever answer is given, two further questions follow. How certain is one of one's opinion? What are its moral implications? The first question is important because it poses the question of doubt of conscience. Is one obliged to treat a doubtful human person as if it were or were not a person? We will return to that question shortly.

If one is confident that the developing embryo becomes a person at some time after fertilisation, what follows from that? It might be judged that the developing embryo should be treated as a human person, even before it is one. Those who argue for this sometimes quote the early Christian writer Tertullian, who said that he is man who will be a man. In short, the question of stages of development may be taken to be of theoretical interest only, and to have no practical importance. Given the importance of human life, this must always be a respectable position and not lightly dismissed.

On the other hand, the absoluteness of this judgment might be mitigated by granting that the need to save the life of the mother would be sufficient justification for permitting the termination of pregnancy before the time of hominisation (becoming a human person). Or one might argue in favour of permitting termination of embryonic life to protect other important values, of less value than human life.

One might go further and permit scientific research which would endanger the embryo before hominisation, on the grounds that the life of an embryo is of less value, before that time, than the value of the fruits of well-intentioned experiments.

Each of these views could be defended by Catholic writers without obvious rational inconsistency, though those outlined in the last two paragraphs are at variance with official Catholic teaching.

But what is the position of someone who argues that ensoulment or hominisation takes place at a later time than fertilisation, but who is only ready to give this opinion probability rather than certainty? Is one entitled to act as though the embryo was not yet a person? Traditionally moral theologians have taught that one should not act when in doubt about the morality of one's action. The doubt should be settled before acting, otherwise one indicates an unconcern for moral goodness. But in the case we are considering the doubt cannot be settled. What should be done in such a case? A solution proposed in the middle ages for such a dilemma is that known as tutiorism. This required that if there was any doubt that an act was morally licit one should not act, even though the reasons which could be adduced in favour of one's liberty to act outweighed those against. The system of tutiorism was rejected in the Church as being unreasonably restrictive of freedom and burdensome to consciences. But until this day authors teach that there are cases in which the safest course should be taken even though there may be good reasons for favouring its opposite. One such case is relevant to our discussion. If a human life is at stake then the safest means of protecting it must be used. In effect the Sacred Congregation of the Doctrine of the Faith, in the text which was quoted earlier, uses a tutiorist argument. We cannot know whether the early embryo is ensouled so we must act on the presumption that it is, lest we risk killing a human being.

Once tutiorism had been rejected as a solution to the majority of cases other systems were suggested. After several hundred years of debate it can be stated with some confidence that a system known as probabilism is safe. According to this system, in practice, if there is an objectively doubtful obligation there can be no certain subjective obligation. In short, if in doubt, one is free to follow whichever course of action is thought good and acceptable, even though good arguments could be adduced in favour of an alternative.

In a complex and careful article in *Theological Studies*, Carol A Tauer argues that the Sacred Congregation is mistaken in its belief that a tutiorist system must be followed in decisions concerning the human embryo.[11] She acknowledges that if the presence of a soul were a question of fact which could, in principle, be empirically verifiable, then one would have to follow the tutiorist solution. There would be no doubt about which moral principle applied. It would be that which forbade direct attacks on innocent human life. The doubt would be about whether there was an innocent human life present. But, she argues, the doubt is not about fact, but about theory. For, as the Congregation admits, the matter can never be settled. She contends that the Catholic tradition would not have solved a doubt of theory by a tutiorist solution. It would have permitted probabilist solutions. If she is right it would follow that, if one were confident in one's own mind that the early human embryo did not have a human soul (and a number of Catholic philosophers and theologians think this even though they would acknowledge that the matter is not certain) then one might act as though it did not have a soul. One might be willing to sacrifice it to secure values which were judged to outweigh that of an unensouled embryo. One might even justify experiments on them of the sort forbidden by the Pope.

Conclusion

Official Catholic teaching requires that human life be protected from conception onwards. This is in line with a tradition going back almost to the beginning of the life of the Church. But at one period in that history there were theologians who thought the ban on direct abortion need not be absolute. Once again, in our day, there are those who suggest that ensoulment comes late and therefore the human embryo need not be given absolute protection from its very beginning. The recent instruction from the Sacred Congregation for the Doctrine of the Faith indicates that the official teaching authority of the Church is determined in its rejection of these opinions.

References

1 John R Connery SJ. *Abortion and the development of the Roman Catholic perspective.* Loyola University Press, 1977.

2 Pourquois l'eglise ne peut accepter l'avortement. *Documentation Catholique*, 70, 1973: pp 4–5. English translation: *The Pope speaks*, 17, 1973: pp 333–335.

3 Richard McCormick SJ. The abortion dossier. *Theological Studies*, 34, 1974: pp 312–359.

4 The Catholic Archbishops of Great Britain. *Abortion and the right to live*, 1980. CTS S345.

5 *See* 4 above: paragraph 12.

6 Sacred Congregation for the Doctrine of the Faith. *Declaratio de abortu procurato*, AA/LXVI, 1974: 730–747, p 738.

7 *See* 4 above: paragraph 21.

8 Pope John Paul II. *Ad eos qui conventui de biologiae experimentis in Vaticana Civitate habito interfuere*, 23 October 1982. AAS 75, 1983: part I, p 37.

9 Congregation for the Doctrine of the Faith. *Instruction on respect for human life in its origin and on the dignity of procreation*. 1987.

10 *In vitro fertilisation and public policy*. Catholic Information Services, 1983: p 8.

11 Carol A Tauer. The tradition of probabilism and the moral status of the early embryo. *Theological Studies*, 45, 1984: pp 3–33.

9

THE ANIMATION TRADITION IN THE LIGHT OF CONTEMPORARY PHILOSOPHY

Peter Byrne

My concern in this chapter is the same as that which pre-occupies a number of my fellow contributors to this volume. It centres on the question: how can we decide whether research involving the manipulation and possible destruction of human embryos is licit? I shall attempt to answer this question through an exploration of the contemporary relevance of the centuries-old teaching on the delayed animation or ensoulment of the human embryo and offer some comment on my fellow contributors' arguments as I do so. A considerable amount of stage-setting is needed, however, before the animation tradition is discussed directly.

The question of whether research on embryos is licit will only arise with some of the procedures associated with *in vitro* fertilisation (IVF) and contemporary embryology. The careful observation of embryonic growth, the intelligent variation of methods of culture and storage, and so on, will be part of the normal practice of the responsible development of IVF as a means of overcoming infertility and yet may involve embryos whose future destiny is implantation into a woman and development into a child in experimental procedures. The moral question broached in this paper will only raise its head where experimental procedures are undertaken outside any such context, where the embryo's future is deliberately disregarded as part of the research or where indeed the nature of the research procedure is incompatible with the embryo having a future. The majority of the research procedures mentioned in chapter 3 involve damage or destruction to the embryos used in them. Here there is room for the embryo's interests to be seen to clash with those of others and thus for us to ask if its interests can be set aside in the light of competing claims. We seek to know if it makes sense to think of the embryo as having an individual good and, if it has, whether the good can easily be seen as subservient to other goods.

Having got thus far we may think it impossible to proceed without deciding directly upon the moral status of the embryo which is in turn linked by a series of seemingly inevitable steps to deciding whether the embryo is a person. But it is worth pausing at this point to see if there is not some way of avoiding these linked decisions. For some maintain that these questions are rationally undecidable in the light of the seemingly intractable disagreement they provoke. If there is even a hint of truth in such scepticism, we are bound to consider whether indirect ways of settling the licitness of embryo research have any cogency. I call such methods of reasoning 'indirect' because they offer some way of determining whether embryo research is licit without deciding upon the possibly undecidable question: 'is a wrong done *to the embryo* in such research?'.

Among indirect means of deciding the acceptability of embryo research, appeal to consequences and shared moral feelings might be considered. The consequences for social and family life for certain types of imagined research (for example, that directed towards sex selection unrelated to inherited sex-linked disorders or other forms of selective breeding) may indeed be disquieting. And embryo research may in general provoke a sense of moral outrage in the public at large. In neither case, however, do we seem to have anything that could bear decisively on the question at issue. The appeal to consequences as I have described it is inevitably selective in its implications. If there are some possible types of research with harmful consequences, they should be controlled or banned. The licitness of research in general remains untouched, unless we are to be influenced by the defeatist argument that, if something *can* be abused for some ends, it *will* be abused regardless of our vigilance. The Chief Rabbi, in his contribution to this volume, makes much of the harmful consequences for the institution of marriage of some possibilities in embryology and the treatment of infertility.[1] These deserve to be taken seriously while the institution of marriage remains something that our society wishes to preserve and foster. However, even he is not against *all* forms of embryological research and thus recognises that no general bar or cut-off point emerges from these considerations. Appeal to feelings is likewise indecisive. This is partly because they have weight only when considered in the context of other moral considerations, but also because they are less trustworthy the further they are removed from everyday moral experience. This is why I would give weight to a general repugnance at killing babies in considering the morality of infanticide, but be more cautious in weighing any alleged general repugnance towards research on embryos. Few have any experience of a human embryo; few indeed know of its appearance and constitution. Is not repugnance, then, directed towards the unknown?

II

I have not considered by any means all the indirect considerations that might be brought to bear on the question of the licitness of embryo research. Let us suppose for the sake of argument that no such indirect considerations bear decisively on the question. Are we not in that case driven to take up the seemingly insoluble matter of if and when the embryo is a person? Not necessarily, for it might be thought that the moral status of the embryo could be settled without concluding that it was a person. Even if the matter of its personhood were ignored or determined in the negative, other ways of deciding its moral status, and thus commenting directly on the licitness of embryo research, are available.

One such alternative method would be a simple utilitarianism which eschewed the 'metaphysical' question of the attainment of personhood in favour of the 'scientific' question of when the embryo acquired sentience. Some will argue that while the former question cannot be decided with certainty, the latter can. Before the embryo is sentient no tangible harm can be done to it by any form of experimental manipulation; after it becomes sentient there is a clear way of judging the moral rectitude of modes of treating it in the balance of pleasure and pain these bring. Whether any view of the ethics of embryo research as naive as this has ever been seriously propounded I cannot say. Its weakness as a way of dodging the question of personhood has been well brought out by John Marshall in this volume. He notes that it provides no check at all on the licitness of research as long as that research is on pre-sentient or anaesthetised embryos.[2] Such a conclusion amounts to abandoning the moral enquiry altogether, so feeble is it. If the only moral principal we can appeal to in these matters is 'cause no pain', the development of anaesthetics for embryos (or fetuses) will remove any force it has. Only if the attainment of sentience is linked to something else (like a theory of personhood) could it avoid the moral simplicity of saying that anything is licit as long as it causes no pain. But any more sophisticated way of using the fact of sentience in this area will inevitably take us back into deeper philosophical waters, because it will be linked to a theory of a richer sort about why sentient creatures should have a special dignity. Utilitarianism applied to the ethics of treating embryos is not a way of avoiding philosophical debate on the status of embryonic life but the conclusion of such debate.

One may glean a different and more sophisticated way of avoiding decision on the question 'when does the embryo become a person?' from Professor Ian Kennedy's writings on this subject.[3] Even if the embryo is not a person the fact that it is an example of human reproductive tissue, and the fact that it has the potential to develop into something that is a person, force the conclusion, according to Kennedy, that research on embryos is never morally permissible. These facts jointly show that the embryo has a special status or worth that may be recognised without agreement on the more abstruse matter of when personhood is acquired.

One of my worries abouth this line of reasoning rests in the manner in which it appeals to our sense of moral repugnance to support the conclusion that we are forced to regard research on the potential human as always wrong. Moreover, the facts about embryos are shared by the unfertilised ovum as well. The special status accruing to the embryo from these facts cannot therefore be different in kind (though it may be different in degree) from that possessed by the ovum. If this be so, it is hard to see how this status could block, once and for all, the sacrifice of embryos in the service of other important human interests – such as research into the prevention of serious diseases. We do not seem to have in these considerations anything that would completely block means-end reasoning about the use of embryos, only some facts which demand that any ends for which the embryo is sacrificed will have to be sufficiently cogent.

The facts pointed to by Kennedy explain why certain ways of creating and/or using embryos give us qualms of conscience quite apart from whether we think the embryo is yet a person. Potential personhood and the obvious connection with human reproduction mean that how we treat embryos is importantly connected with our attitudes to humanity in general, regardless of our views about embryos and personhood. I catch an awareness of this dimension of our treatment of embryos in the Chief Rabbi's criticism of the creation of embryos purely for experimental purposes or for the supply of organs for transplant. This, he contends, will lead to the mechanisation of human procreation and the consequent degradation of all human life.[4] This is an important dimension to the ethics of embryo research which deserves to be taken seriously. But again I conclude that it does not place a bar on research as such; it merely points to the need for restraint and limitation in its pursuit.

III

Having examined some alternative approaches I now return to the question of whether, and if so when, the embryo is a person, because only a decision about the personhood of the embryo will bring any clear sense of the obligations owed to it. Only the ascription of personhood at some point in its development will provide a decisive block upon means-end reasoning with respect to its treatment. It is of persons that we say that they are never to be treated merely as means but always to be respected as ends in themselves.

The above formula about means and ends owes much, of course, to Kant's moral philosophy with its famous injunction always to treat humanity, whether in one's own person or in others', as an end in itself.[5] The meaning of Kant's formula is connected with his belief that each being who is a person is an instance of practical rationality, a being with desires and interests and the capacity to reason how best to fulfil those desires and interests and to act accordingly. When we act in relation to such a being we are to respect his ends even while we try to pursue our own; that is, we must not hinder, and indeed ought to promote, that being's capacity to pursue his own ends. His ends therefore provide checks on how we attain our own, rather than being at the mercy of the efficient pursuit of our goals. In the Kantian tradition, then, persons are the source of a unique constraint on the efficient attainment of goals. The exception to this constraint arises when the ends of one whom we recognise to be a person themselves threaten another's ends, as in the case of a thief or murderer; justice then demands that we set aside some of the ends of a rational creature.

This Kantian mode of thinking has provided much of the basis for contemporary moral philosophy's account of the peculiar worth and importance of persons. The mention of justice in my description of it leads into another way of characterising the moral nature of personhood. This is implicit in much of our ordinary thought about the treatment of persons and again points to the importance of the notion of personhood in the embryo debate.

We discover this mode of characterisation when we say that it is to persons, and only to persons, that the notion of just/unjust treatment applies. There are sources of moral demands and constraints other than justice, such as benevolence and courage. Justice is that virtue or sphere of moral constraint concerned with giving what is owing or due to those we encounter in moral life. To kill an animal while causing it suffering is wrong because cruelty is wrong. To kill a human infant, even painlessly, is wrong because a wrong is thereby done to the infant. An act of injustice has been committed in the second case but not in the first. The second example of killing violates what is owing and due to the victim, namely respect and care for his life. So it is an instance of unjust killing or murder. What is not a person cannot be murdered, though in certain circumstances it may be wrong to kill it.[6] The strikingness of such vegetarian slogans as 'meat eating is murder' depends on their oddity. This dimension to the appraisal of our treatment of persons produces constraints on our actions which go beyond guarding against the infliction of pain or distress. Justice places checks on the attainment of our ends that transcend the dimensions of kindness and/or cruelty. In reflection on what is due and owing to another person we realise that he is not to be used as an unwitting tool in the achievement of our goals if we thereby hamper his own future development and prospects. This is so regardless of whether he is aware of the effects of our actions in a painful way or not.

It is a significant advance in our own age that general moral thought has come to accept that being a human is a sufficient, though not of course a necessary, condition for enjoying the status of a person. We would not normally insist on the presence of extra conditions – such as being also white, male and Anglo-Saxon. Though there may be other ways of enjoying this status, sharing in human nature is in itself sufficient to give someone this status.[7] In this recognition lies the possibility of finding personhood in the prenatal human organism and thus of finding a firmly grounded check to means-ends reasoning at some point in prenatal development.

Despite the moral agreement noted above it is depressing to have to note an influential body of opinion in contemporary moral philosophy that does hold that some extra conditions, over and above mere humanity, *are* required for the attainment of personhood. A brief consideration of the line of thought will help to bring out further the basis for the ascription of personhood and some of the detailed principles that need to be employed in thinking about the status of the embryo.

A work such as Jonathan Glover's *Causing Death and Saving Lives*[8] uses a notion of personhood similar to Kant's, linking personhood to the exercise of rational thought and action. This notion goes back to the classical sources of the animation tradition and was given definitive expression in Boethius's definition of the person: 'The individual substance of rational nature'.[9] Glover and those who think like him argue in effect that rational nature can only bring enhanced moral status if it can be expressed in the present (in such things as self-conscious desires for long-term ends). So humanity turns out not to be a sufficient condition for personhood after all, since only those human beings with certain present qualities turn out to be persons. The way is then open to raise doubts about, even to deny, the status of infants, mentally defective individuals, and certain old people, as persons. The radical moral conclusions which may follow from this are indicated in Glover's statement that there are no direct reasons why infanticide is wrong. Leaving aside our feelings and provided that we inflict no pain, babies are replaceable. They may be killed with moral propriety if new ones are produced to replace the old.[10] Such conclusions are another indication of the link between the category of personhood and the unique constraints proceeding from justice.

The unwholesomeness of the conclusions described above may be considered sufficient reason for rejecting the line of thought from which they derive. Consideration of three related notions can add further weight to the refusal to give up the belief that being a human is sufficient for being a person. These three notions are potentiality, nature and history. Each is vital in understanding the animation tradition and in judging whether the concept of personhood can be taken back to prenatal life.

Consider first the notion of potentiality. There is a tendency in the school of thought, of which Glover is so clearly a representative, to award the status of personhood only to those entities that display in the present the qualities of a rational nature. But even this school of thought must allow some elasticity in this, for it will not deny personhood to an otherwise normal adult who is asleep and thus displaying no qualities of rational thought or action. Such a person has the present capacity for these qualities even without their actual display. Something weaker than present capacity is required to cope with another obvious case. A normal adult who has lost consciousness through accident or illness will still be regarded as a person even though he neither displays nor has the present capacity to display rational life. Such a person may require active and massive help by outside agencies before recovering the ability to exercise these powers, but is still to be accounted a person because the fundamental biological structures on which these powers rest are unimpaired or, if damaged, repairable. Let us say that such a person has a real potential to display rational powers. If we are prepared to allow a set of potentialities to count as sufficient for personhood, there seems to be no reason why we should deny that human infants are persons.[11] Have they not real potentials for the display of rational powers?

Glover's answer to the line of argument about potentiality advanced here is that if mere possibility can be sufficient for the award of personhood, any preceding stage in the development of a human being should be awarded this status, since in all the possibility of developing into something with the relevant capacities and endowments is prefigured. On this ground personhood could be granted to the ovum, for it is possible that it may become something with the capacities of a person. This is an attempt to reduce the case for granting personhood to infants to an absurdity, suggesting that the criterion of potentiality is so inclusive as to have no substance at all.[12] In reply an attempt must be made to distinguish the genuine potentiality the infant has for exercising rational nature from anything so weak as a

94

mere possibility. The possibility that an ovum will become a person depends upon external intervention (fertilisation) which at the same time leads to the transformation of its inner nature and biological constitution. It has to become a radically different kind of organism if this possibility is to be realised. Yet, while a new-born infant depends upon many external stimuli and much nurture to realise its potential to display the capacities belonging to a rational existence, these external influences will not transform it into a different kind of creature. They will instead awaken and develop tendencies already latent in its constitution. It is already fashioned so that these tendencies are inherent in it. So something substantial is said when it is affirmed that the infant has real potential for the exercise of the powers of a rational life. The ground for granting personhood has not been weakened to the point where it loses sufficient power of discrimination.

The force of the concept of potentiality is strengthened when we reflect on the associated notion of nature. Boethius's definition tells us that a person is an individual substance of rational nature. Now, that something has a rational nature does not entail that it must, in the present, display or possess in a realised form the capacities of a rational life. The unconscious adult, the infant and the aged comatose or non-compos patient all possess the nature of rational beings. They share in rational nature even though they have lost or not yet acquired the present ability to express that nature.[13] They have the constitution of beings of their kind who are able to display the qualities of a rational existence even though the expression of this nature is impaired or undeveloped. It is the first emergence and eclipse of this inner nature that set the proper boundaries to the ascription of the concept of personhood to human beings. These boundaries in the case of human persons are the same as those for humanity itself, since to be human is, among other things, to be an animal having rational nature. This is true even though no human being displays this nature in a realised way through all his life and even though some, alas, never do.

95

Boethius's definition provides a route into the final concept that needs to be considered at this stage of the argument – history. One thing that can be drawn from this definition is that valuing rational nature is not a matter of valuing the human being as a mere occasion for the display or existence of rationality. We value the substance which possesses this nature. By 'individual substance' Boethius may have in mind particularly a being with a history. If the individual substance is the object of respect, it is to be respected throughout its history and not merely during those times when it is displaying most fully or clearly the qualities of personhood that are the grounds for our respect. To adopt this latter stance *is* to value the enduring being as merely the occasion for the qualities.[14] If we rightly refuse this occasionalism, we must respect all stages in the continuing history of that being, including those stages which come before and after the actual display of rational nature. Thus we value the enduring individual at his beginning and end, not merely in his prime.

IV

I hope that I have offered, so far, some substantial considerations in favour of a number of conclusions that are relevant and helpful in deciding upon the moral status of the embryo and upon the licitness of embryo research. These conclusions draw support from strands of reflection in the contemporary philosophy though, as I have indicated, there is by no means unanimous agreement. They include the following. (1) The concept of personhood is vital in describing the moral status of human beings. It is therefore important to trace the beginnings of its applicability if an assured answer to the question of the licitness of embryo research is to be reached; otherwise we are forced to rely on a number of indirect considerations which cannot provide a definitive check to means-end reasoning. (2) There is reason to make humanity a sufficient condition for the attainment of personhood. (3) There are grounds, through reflection on the concepts of potentiality, nature and the history of an individual, for tracing humanity and therefore personhood to new-born life. But if we can trace personhood back to infancy by these means we should be able to trace it back to at least some stages of prenatal life as well. For the sense in which a new-born human infant possesses real potential for rational life, or has the nature of a rational being or is one stage in the history of an 'individual substance' is also true of the prenatal being for at least much of its history. These various foundations of personhood are ultimately dependent upon the infant's biological constitution, and the biological constitution of the infant is obviously rooted in that of the embryo/fetus. So that if personhood is awarded to the infant on these grounds it must, to be consistent, be granted to at least some stages of prenatal life.

In recent publications, both Gordon Dunstan and John Mahoney[15,16,17] have reminded us of the antiquity and extent of a tradition of thinking about the moral status of the embryo that goes back at least to Aristotle and is supported by much of Christian theology until at least the nineteenth century. This tradition is based on the doctrine of the delayed animation or ensoulment of the embryo/fetus. Despite the difference in terminology, this doctrine is strikingly in accord with some of the lines of thought from contemporary philosophy that I have drawn out. The theological/metaphysical side of the speculation about the point of ensoulment among medieval writers was kept in check by a reading of Aristotle. The key to his thought on the status of the embryo was the belief that the embryo only became informed and animated on acquiring an intellectual soul at 40–80 days after conception (depending upon the sex of the embryo – compare *Leviticus* 12:1–5). As Dunstan and Mahoney note, acquiring an intellectual soul is linked in Aristotle's discussion to the biological development of the embryo and so we have here significant historical support for some of the ideas developed in this chapter; that is, we see the value of human beings in their possession of a rational nature and this nature can be traced back to prenatal life because it is based on a biological foundation

97

which is laid down in a substantial way before birth. The idea that comes from the animation tradition that this laying down is not complete at conception adds in an important way to anything argued so far, for if it is taken up it will lead to the conclusion that decisive objections to means-ends reasoning with respect to the embryo/fetus will only arise some time after conception. Thus it may be concluded that embryo research is an open possibility. Dunstan and Mahoney both note that, influenced by the belief in delayed animation, the Church taught for centuries that to destroy an unformed fetus was not to commit homicide and therefore not to commit murder. Murder would fall under the absolute bar of 'Do not do evil that good may come of it'. In religious tradition this bar applies to the case of murder because of the content of *Exodus* 23:7: ' . . . the innocent and the righteous slay thou not'.

The animation tradition offers an evolutionary view of the status of the embryo/fetus. In considering what can be said in favour of this view the first point to note is its coherence with the thought that moral status depends upon the acquisition of a nature or a set of potentialities that must be biologically grounded. It seems reasonable to suppose that if the biological constitution of the embryo/ fetus develops, so must its moral status. Another general argument for an evolutionary view of the moral status of the embryo/fetus can be gathered from L W Sumner.[18] Most would accept that the peculiar moral standing of persons does not attach to ova or spermatozoa but does to new-born infants. The gap between the moral status of infants and ova must be bridged at some point between fertilisation and birth. The moral standing in which we are interested must be acquired during the life of the embryo/fetus. There are then three possibilities. (1) This moral standing is acquired at the point of fertilisation itself and thus is enjoyed by the embryo/fetus throughout gestation. (2) This moral standing is acquired at birth, and prior to it the embryo/fetus does not enjoy the status of a person. (3) This moral standing is present before birth but arises with biological development after fertilisation and so is not present from the very beginning of embryonic life. Moralists of course disagree about which of these three is the most plausible but, as Sumner notes, there is an element of common sense in preferring (3). For both (1) and (2) seem wedded to the paradox that the enormous biological changes during the course of fetal and embryonic life are of little or no relevance to the question of the moral status of the embryo/fetus. It is surely implausible to suppose that the whole moral question rests on what happens to one or other of the extreme points between which massive biological development occurs.

Considerations have been given in favour of the idea that the moral status of personhood should be taken into prenatal life. Further considerations can be offered in favour of the distinguishing feature of possibility (3) – the belief that only post-fertilisation development within prenatal life gives an adequate foundation for personhood. Chief among these might be the fact of the undifferentiated nature of the embryonic matter in the days immediately following conception. If this matter is not even differentiated into that which will become the fetus and that which will develop into the placenta, it is hard to see how there is sufficient foundation for the ascription of the beginning of personal, human life. The concepts of human nature, of real potentials for a certain kind of life and of the beginnings of the history of an individual substance do not get a grip until the achievement of significant steps in the differentiation of the matter of the embryo.

The well-known and much discussed possibility of monozygotic twinning provides a further reason for adopting conclusion (3) on the status of the embryo/fetus. It is linked especially to the idea that a personal being must be one with a history. This in turn entails that a person must have a unique, stable and enduring existence. If we consider the possibility that up to about 14 days after fertilisation the embryo can split and even re-unite again it is plausible to conclude that it is not yet the historical being that a person by definition is. There is not sufficient stability in the early embryo to count it as a human being.

John Mahoney sums up the line of argument just advanced as follows:

> ... the major element of the argument lies in the inherent possibility for twinning and combination which exists at least up to nidation. Underlying this approach appears to be the realisation that some biological stability in the organism is essential for its individuality to be established, and that without this stable individuation of the organism one cannot begin to speak of a human individual.[19]

If these arguments are judged cogent they will lead to the conclusion that the embryo does not have the unique moral status of a person in at least the first two weeks of its existence. Non-beneficial research on embryos will then be an arguable possibility during this period (balancing the ends of research against the kinds of consideration discussed briefly in section II above). Some may wish to extend this period during which research is an arguable possibility if they interpret the need for the matter of the embryo to have a human-like form and differentiation in a certain way. The rational nature of the human infant, its real potentials for rational life, depend essentially upon its possession of brain and nervous system. It could therefore be argued that embryos may properly be treated as less than persons up to the point where brain and nervous system come to be laid down as differentiated types of tissue, and this may take the limit of research into the second month after fertilisation. Such an extension would not be granted out of any concern to use sentience as a major criterion, but rather because of the need to see evidence of the emergence of the specifically human biological foundation of person-hood in the development of the embryo. Most of the research possibilities mentioned in chapter 3 would then appear to be open, provided that they did not involve the destruction of embryonic/fetal life after the second month of gestation, and granted that the medical goals behind them were judged sufficiently weighty.

100

V

The argument of sections III and IV is the crux of this paper. It is worthwhile offering a summary of it and further clarification of some of the concepts it employs, and particularly of how notions like potentiality and constitution are used in it.

The definition of 'person' used in my argument is Boethius's ('the individual substance of rational nature'). The limits of personhood are explored by reference to three subordinate notions – substance, nature and potentiality – and with the aim of commenting on two important questions. (1) Is being a human being sufficient for being a person? (2) Can the attributes of personhood be taken back into prenatal life?

The concept of potentiality is the source of *one* reason for answering the first question in the affirmative. Rationality in a creature consists in the possession of certain powers, including those for self-conscious experience, memory, deliberative choice, drawing inferences and being aware of long-term goals. In ordinary language and law we speak of persons who are not exercising such powers in the present and who do not have them as realised capacities in the present. There is sense in saying that children or the seriously ill are persons because, among other things, they have real potential for exercising the powers of personhood. That is, they have enough of the causal basis for the enjoyment and exercise of such powers, even if that basis is not being stimulated at present, or the ability to exercise these powers is damaged, impaired or not fully developed, or if all the causal basis is not yet perfected.

'Potential' talk assimilates a being not at present exercising rational capacities to one who is, only if it is closely analogous to talk of a thing's tendencies, as opposed to talk of what a thing could be transformed into by external causal factors. A crude illustration of the difference would be this: compare 'A young tree has the potential to bear fruit' with 'The bricks and mortar are potentially a house'. I associate myself with one way of analysing power-statements in the philosophy of science and adapt talk of real potentials to that. Just as with real potentials things and materials can have powers when they are not exercising them. The distinction between things which have different powers does not necessarily lie in what *will* happen to them or in what they *will* do. For it is only a contingent fact, if it is true at all, that their differing powers will be exercised. So it is with things which have different potentials. Things with different powers are different *in the present* because the basis for their differing powers must be a distinction in inner constitution, that is, in the intrinsic causal factors of their make-up. The same applies to things with different potentials.[20] Talk of something's real potential is not just talk about what it could be made into in the course of time, but about its inherent tendencies as these are determined by its constitution. Talk of 'X's real potential to V' can only assimilate X to things which actually V if such talk is based on the presence in X, at least in some form, of the causal basis for V-ing.

What is the causal basis for the actions of rational substance in the case of humanity? It is the possession of a human nature, including genetic endowment of a certain sort, and a particular form of anatomy, physiology and histology. We have real potentials for such acts at the start of human life only when we have the beginnings of the assemblage of such a causal basis in the infant or the fetus or the embryo. It is the clear absence of such a basis in the ovum which makes me say that it and the infant have a different constitution.

The main problems that could arise with my appeal to potentiality and constitution appear to be as follows:

1   There is a tendency in biology to identify constitution with genetic endowment.

2   There are links in the constitution of the ovum, early embryo, late embryo, fetus, infant. There have to be such links otherwise these would not count as different stages of the one process of metamorphosis.

3   Uncontroversial judgment as to the presence of enough of the constitution of a human being sufficient to have real potentials of the requisite sort is impossible.

102

The case offered in sections III and IV is for concluding that we could not have the real potential for personhood in an embryonic human substance unless it had the genetic endowment of a human being; it had achieved the stability of a human being; and its matter had begun to have the significant differentiation of the matter of a human being (that is, the beginnings of organogenesis had occurred). With these three conditions the embryonic human organism has begun to have the constitution of a human being, in the relevant sense of 'constitution' – the sense determined by my argument and not necessarily that currently used by biologists.

VI

The arguments of sections IV and V are intended to amount to a sketch of a case for a graduated approach to the licitness of embryo research. These arguments allow that there could be ends which outweigh the harm of destruction of the embryo up to 14 days of development and, perhaps, beyond. But after some recognisably early point in embryonic development, research is to be governed by much the same criteria as apply to experiments on infants. More specifically, most of the research possibilities mentioned in chapter 3 would appear to be open if they did not involve the destruction of embryonic/fetal life after the second month of gestation. The arguments offered for these conclusions are based on a moral philosophy which may of course be rejected by many. But even those who accept the general approach to moral standing which lies behind it might have reason to doubt the conclusions reached. Let me note and discuss two objections that could come from one who thought that a graduated approach was wrong because the embryo enjoys full moral standing from conception onwards.

Such an objector might first query my attempt to show that there is some genuine historical consensus among the makers of the Western moral tradition in favour of a developmental view. Following Dunstan, I have tried to insinuate such an opinion as part of an attempt to show that in historical thought and contemporary moral philosophy there may be a basis for resolving the question of the status of the human embryo. An objector could argue that regardless of any speculations about delayed ensoulment, the Christian Church has always taught that destruction of embryonic life is a sin regardless of the stage of development the embryo has reached. The differences in canon law over the penalties and penances attaching to the destruction of the unborn at different stages of growth are unimportant in this context.[21]

What this objection certainly shows is that it is wrong to appeal to moral tradition to demonstrate that there has long been support for the specific conclusion that research on early embryos is morally an open question. It would be anachronistic to say that the modes of thought Dunstan and Mahoney document either directly support or directly condemn the types of procedures now called 'embryo research'. The context of what is under discussion today is different from the kinds of interference with unborn life considered by moralists and lawyers many centuries ago. We can gain from the animation tradition a point of agreement on a theoretical matter and this point can be made to bear moral fruit if we extrapolate from it in the present. This extrapolation can gain some general support from the moral tradition if we repeat a point made earlier, namely that the tradition did not regard destruction of the unformed embryo as murder and did not therefore place this act among those that could never be done regardless of objective, end or circumstances. Even to characterise this act as one of homicide would not have placed it in this category since the notion of a justifiable homicide was allowed in various forms; but the tradition does not count early destruction as homicide and it would have been totally inconsistent with the speculative part of the animation tradition to have counted it as such.

A defender of the notion that full moral standing associated with personhood must be granted immediately upon fertilisation will also wish to press the case for saying that the coming together of the genetic endowment of a human individual at that point should be taken as the true beginning of an 'individual substance of rational nature'. The genetic endowment of the individual is, leaving aside nurture and stimuli, the most fundamental factor behind subsequent development and thus deserves to be identified as the true, unchanging biological constitution that is the foundation of personal life.

My reply to this point will largely have to consist of contentions already made. While acknowledging the importance of genetic endowment as an underlying causal factor, I would have to stress again the great changes needed in the constitution of the being immediately in possession of this endowment (the very early embryo) before it can be taken to be a human individual. The points about the differention and stability of the later embryo already made are meant to show that it, and the subsequent fetus and infant, are different in nature and constitution in a morally relevant way from the very early embryo – a morally relevant way because they are related to the concept of a person.

Supposing this reply is accepted as sufficient, a further question can be pressed: if a reading of the concept of personhood is adopted that looks forward from the mere coming together of genetic endowment, can it in consistency stop short of the substantial completion of fetal development? It is claimed that even a two-months embryo lacks a full human-like anatomy and physiology and has not yet acquired anything like the full range of organs and tissue types of a human being. Judged from the standpoint of anatomy, physiology and histology, does it not make better sense to deny that the embryo/fetus is a human being (as opposed to a human becoming) until at least some six months into gestation?[22] I have of course wanted to look back into earlier stages of gestation from that point, not only because to do so is required by any attempt to stay within the animation tradition but also because a developmental view of the embryo/fetus would be uninteresting otherwise. Taking the award of personhood to such a late stage would leave the developmental view totally lacking in moral bite in the context of embryo research. What an objector may wish to know is whether there is any sufficient basis for going back from the last stages of gestation that does not rely on genetic endowment as the link to personhood and does not take us right back to fertilisation.

The Aristotelian bias of my argument leads me to take personhood back into the early weeks of gestation only if biology shows a continuity of constitution between late fetus/new born infant and the embryo at early stages. Genetic endowment will not do because there are great discontinuities apparent between the very early embryo and the developed human organism of late pregnancy despite shared endowment. For all the force of the objection summarised above I see great continuities of inner constitution between the embryo of, say, two months and the viable fetus. For by that stage the embryo has achieved the stability of a unique individual and is undergoing a process whereby the beginnings of the organs and physiological systems of the human being are being laid down. From the eighth week onwards the continuity between earlier and later stages is clearly marked: as Mary Seller notes in her chapter, development thereafter largely consists of the growth and maturation of organs and systems which have already been laid down during the embryonic period.[23]

VII

The case for a developmental view of the status of the human embryo offered here is guided by the thought that there can be a reasoned answer to the question it addresses and therefore to the linked question of the licitness of embryo research. These are matters on which argument is appropriate and can aim, like all argument, at common assent.

This is not to say that the moral status of the embryo is a plain fact which can be read off from incontrovertible data. The reasoning possible in this area seems to be parallel to those other cases where the application of a concept to a fresh or problematic instance is being decided upon. The freshness of the instance prevents us from reading off the answer to the question of whether the concept applies from some existing and non-controversial rule. We are to a degree extending the concept in applying it to this case. But our decision that it does or does not apply to this instance need not be the expression of an ungrounded choice. There can be a logic to the extension of concepts. Whether the concept is to be extended can be decided by reference to its established sense and what fits in with this. Consideration of the animation tradition can help bring home the point that the relevant concept in this case – the concept of personhood – is one with an established sense and is not to be remade anew and arbitrarily.

The fact that there appears to be an element of decision in the resolution of the question of the moral status of the embryo need embarrass us no more than the corresponding element of decision in, say, the legal question of whether some hitherto unexamined type of act is or is not negligent. Decision on the extension of a concept need not spell the end of argument or the search for common assent. However, it must be admitted that there are some peculiar difficulties in the question of the moral status of the embryo which go beyond the normal problems encountered in discussing the proper extension of concepts. I shall now consider some of these special problems.

One arises through lack of any complete agreement on which concept and its extension the matter of the embryo's status is to fall under. Some of the philosophers influenced by Utilitarianism in our century would deny that questions of moral standing are best settled by considering the proper extension of the concept of personhood. They might regard some such concept as that of a being with interests as more appropriate. So here is a prior theoretical issue concerning how the question is to be approached. This need not destroy the possibility of a reasoned decision on the matter, since such theoretical questions are themselves the subject of rational discussion, but it does increase the degree of difficulty in presenting any final view as a compelling outcome of argument.

A further important problem arises through the tendency of central concepts like personhood to reveal themselves on analysis to have a number of interpretations, the consequence of their being the subject of competing theories. There may be no single, unambiguous sense to appeal to in deciding upon their extension. Some of these interpretations might make my pursuit of the biological underpinnings of the extension of the concept quite inappropriate. This fact is clearly illustrated in the Chief Rabbi's description of the rabbinic notion that the full status of personhood is not acquired until the emergence of the fetus from the womb. It is the fact of the infant's independent existence of the mother that makes the crucial moral difference on this account and not the degree of its biological development.[24] Speculations about the precise biological affinity between infant and embryo/fetus at earlier stages become irrelevant, as does the animation tradition in which these are rooted. As I understand the Chief Rabbi's views, the licitness of research on the embryo is to be decided by the kinds of considerations mentioned in sections I and II of this chapter (no doubt suitably expanded) and never by speculation about when the embryo becomes a person.

This example from rabbinic thought may, because of the undoubted influence that thought has had upon Western culture, be taken to throw doubt on how far 'we' share an agreed concept of personhood. The revealed basis of the rabbinic doctrine is a reading of passages in *Exodus* in the Hebrew Bible. However, given the disputed character of interpretations of revelation and, more importantly, the widespread rejection of the authority of revelation in secular society, this revealed basis is unlikely to figure much in the moral arguments which hold sway in our society. Expressed independently of its revealed basis the rabbinic doctrine seems to represent what may be called a 'social' theory of personhood, as opposed to the 'substantial' or 'biological' conception of personhood discussed so far. If I were giving expression to this theory independent of its religious setting I would put it thus. What makes something a person is not its nature, rational or otherwise, but its existence as an independent member of an appropriate community – one where certain types of relationship between its members are possible. The human community is such a community and birth into it is therefore sufficient for acquiring the status of personhood. The precise moment of birth may be arbitrary, if it is considered from the standpoint of the biological endowment of the human organism, but personhood does not depend on the details of endowment.

I do not pretend to have presented anything like a full sketch of this different account of what it is to be a person. It may be asked even after so brief an outline whether it does display an alternative concept of personhood or merely another nuance in 'our' single, shared concept. This is the question of whether the social and the substantial theories are or are not reconcilable and complementary. It is important to note in this regard that both will support the belief that infants, the incompetent and the insane are persons, thus making common ground against the trends in contemporary philosophy which limit the award of full moral standing to some favoured class of human beings only. The vital question is whether the achievement of independence outside the womb is taken to be a necessary or a sufficient condition of becoming a person for human beings. If the former, the social and substantial conceptions stand as rivals and a choice has to be made between them in deciding whether or not to trace personhood back into prenatal life. If the latter, then they are complementary and may be used singly and jointly to decide when something is a person.

But now, why is not this final question – of whether independence is necessary or sufficient in the award of personhood – a matter for debate within our concept of a person?

References and notes

1 *See* page 72 of chapter 7.
2 *See* page 60 of chapter 6.

3 *See* I M Kennedy. *The Times*, 26 May 1984.

4 *See* page 9 of *Human fertilisation and embryology: a Jewish view.* London, Office of the Chief Rabbi, 1984.

5 L W Beck (ed) *Groundwork of the metaphysics of morals.* Indianapolis, Bobbs-Merril, 1959: pp 46–47.

6 *See Euthanasia and clinical practice.* London, Linacre Centre, 1982: pp 25–28. These remarks on the status of animals require much fuller support than I am able to offer here.

7 *See* Teresa Iglesias. Social and ethical aspects of IVF. In: *Test tube babies: a Christian view.* London, Unity Press (Order of Christian Unity), 1984: p 72.

8 J Glover. *Causing death and saving lives.* Harmondsworth, Penguin, 1977.

9 Quoted by J Teichman in: The definition of person. *Philosophy*, 60, 236, 1985: p 178.

10 *See* 8 above: pp 139, 159 and 163.

11 *See* P Devine. Abortion, contraception and infanticide. *Philosophy*, 58, 226, 1983: p 516.

12 *See* 8 above: p 122.

13 *See* 9 above: pp 180–182.

14 For this argument *see* 11 above: p 515.

15 G R Dunstan. The moral status of the human embryo: a tradition recalled. *Journal of Medical Ethics*, 10, 1, 1984: pp 38–44. Amplified in chapter 5 of this book.

16 Council for Science and Society. *Human procreation: ethical aspects of the new techniques.* Oxford, Oxford University Press, 1984: pp 5ff.

17 J Mahoney. *Bioethics and belief.* London, Sheed and Ward, 1984: p 56.

18 L W Sumner. *Abortion and moral theory.* Ithica, Cornell University Press, 1981: p 126.

19 *See* 17 above: p 64.

20 *See* R Harre and E H Madden. *Causal powers.* Oxford, Basil Blackwell, 1975: pp 86 and 92.

21 *See* 7 above: p 77.

22 *See* L Becker. Human being: the boundaries of the concept. In: M Cohen, T Nagel and T Scanlon (eds) *Medicine and moral philosphy.* Princeton, Princeton University Press: p 33.

23 *See* p 19 of chapter 2.

24 *See* p 62 of chapter 7.

INDEX

Blackstone, Sir William, 46
Blastocyst, 10
  formation, 18
Blastomeres, formation, 18
Blood disorders, stem cell
  transplants, 29
Blood vessel formation, 19
Boethius, 55, 93, 95, 96, 101
Bone marrow transplants, 29
Brain, formation, and attainment
  of personhood, 100
Brain cell proliferation, 59

Cancer, research into embryonic
  antigens, 28
Canon law, on causing a
  miscarriage, compared with
  common law, 45–6
Canones Hibernenses, 45
Casuistry
  applied to abortion, 77
  definition, 74
Catholic Archbishops of England
  and Wales, 78, 79
Catholic Bishops' Joint
  Committee on Bio-ethical
  Issues, 80
Celtic Penitentials, 45
Central nervous system
  development, 59
    as point beyond which
    research not acceptable, 56
  formation, 19, 49, 100
Cerebral cortex,
  development, 59
Children
  born and raised within
  marriage, 68, 69
  right to identifiable natural
  parents, 73
China, implication of birth
  control programme, 37–8
Christian moral teaching, 10
  no absolute protection for life, 40
  on destruction of embryonic
  life, 104

sources of moral teaching, 75
Chromosome abnormalities at
  conception, 23
  lethality, 24
  major types, 23–4
  research, 23–4
  time of occurrence, 24
Chromosome pairs, genetic
  exchange, 13
Cleavage, 10
Cleaving embryo
  antigens, 28
  moral status, 13
  not yet an individual, 55
  respect due to, 14
Cleft palate, 29
Cloning, 71
Codex Iuris Canonici, 52
Conception
  animation not
  contemporaneous, 98
  as beginning of life, 39–40,
  77–8, 105
Conceptus, 18–19
  sex-determination, 33
Congenital abnormalities, 28
  abortion
    Jewish teaching, 67
  correcting, 70
  determination in
  pregnancy, 33–4
  embryo research, 16
  predicting degree of handicap,
  35
  study of morphogenesis, 28–9
  see also Teratogenesis
Congenital heart defects, 29
Consanguinity, 68
Consent in Medicine, 9
Constantinople, 54
Contraception, 75
  compared with homicide, 77
  forbidden by papal bull, 50
  postcoital, 15, 55
Cryopreservation, 26
  condemned, 80, 81

113

116

potential to become persons, 94–5
status, compared with embryos, 90

Pain
 and licitness of research, 89
 as cut-off point for embryo research, 58–61
 physiological reactions, 58–9
 related to nervous system development, 59–60
 subjectivity, 58
 see also Sentience
Parents, identifiability, 69, 73
Penafort, Raymond de, 45–6
Penances
 graded by fetal age, 45, 46, 50
 for abortion, sterilisation and contraception, 77
Perinatal deaths
 chromosome abnormalities, 23
Persia, 54
Personality, 14
 ethical view of developmental stage, 49
 Henry of Bracton's criteria, 46
 linked to unique individuality, 55
 when achieved, 81
Personhood
 and humanity, 96
 and moral status, 88, 96
 and duties owed to embryo, 90–1
 and rationality, 91
 as bearing legal rights, 14
 at birth, 62, 108
 Boethius's definition, 93, 95, 96, 101
 doubt as to existence, 82
 humanity a condition of, 92–3
 incompatible with possession by another, 37
 Kantian philosophy, 91
 linked to post-fertilisation

development, 99
 moral implications, 12
 of embryo, 14, 88, 97
 regardless of intellectual endowment, 109
 relative to individual history, 96
Philosophic reasoning, 11
Pius IX, Pope, 51, 52, 53–4
Placenta
 formation, 18–19
 see also Trophoblast
Potentiality, 94–5, 96, 101–2
Pregnancy
 estimation of prenatal age, 21
 research into serious conditions, 27
Pregnancy termination, 75
 and sacredness of life, 39
 and time of animation, 78
 as frustration of divine will, 63
 direct and indirect defined, 77
 disposal of embryo of unwanted sex, 34
 during first 40 days, 63–4
 excommunication, 50, 52
 for health of mother, 82
 in Jewish teaching, 70
 in mid-19th century, 51–2
 in rape cases, 15–16
 incidence, 27
 indications, 15
 maternal harm threatened, 35
 method according to pregnancy stage, 28
 research into improved methods, 27–8
Premature labour, causes, 27
Primitive streak, 13
 as point beyond which research not acceptable, 56
 formation, 19
Probabilism, 83–4
Protection of fetus, duty of, 14
Pyruvates, in embryo culture, 22

118